RAND

Governance for Whom and for What

Principles to Guide Health Policy in Miami-Dade County

Catherine A. Jackson, Kathryn Pitkin Derose,
Amanda Beatty

Prepared for Camillus House

RAND Health

The research described in this report was conducted by RAND Health for Community Voices-Miami based at Camillus House.

Library of Congress Cataloging-in-Publication Data

A profile of RAND Health, abstracts of its publications, and ordering information can be found on the RAND Health home page at www.rand.org/health.

Published 2003 by RAND
1700 Main Street, P.O. Box 2138, Santa Monica, CA 90407-2138
1200 South Hayes Street, Arlington, VA 22202-5050
201 North Craig Street, Suite 202, Pittsburgh, PA 15213-1516
RAND URL: http://www.rand.org/
To order RAND documents or to obtain additional information, contact Distribution Services: Telephone: (310) 451-7002; Fax: (310) 451-6915; Email: order@rand.org

Preface

In response to continuing concerns over access to health care for the uninsured, the W. K. Kellogg Foundation in 1998 launched an initiative called "Community Voices." The goal of the initiative is to assist local organizations in strengthening community support services, giving the underserved a voice in the debate over health care access, and identifying ways to meet the needs of those who now receive inadequate health care. One of the Community Voices grants went to Miami, Florida, where it is administered by Camillus House, a Catholic social service agency and health care provider for the homeless.[1] Camillus House asked RAND to participate in the Community Voices–Miami project, to evaluate the five-year effort and to provide technical assistance.

This report is the second of the technical assistance reports produced by RAND for Community Voices. The first report, *Hospital Care for the Uninsured in Miami-Dade County: Hospital Finance and Patient Travel Patterns* (Jackson et al., 2002), analyzed publicly available hospital financial and discharge data to determine whether there was any correlation between the centralized nature of funding for and provision of indigent care in Miami-Dade County and the hospital-care-seeking patterns of Miami-Dade County residents. That analysis showed that the uninsured living in the more-remote areas of the county bypassed more hospitals than did their insured neighbors, creating disparities in geographic access to care.

This study addresses the issue of governance of public funds for health care in Miami-Dade County. The county-run Public Health Trust is currently responsible for operating the county's health care facilities, as well as for developing countywide planning to ensure access to health care for all residents. Over time, this dual mission has introduced challenges to good governance.

The study was conducted by researchers in the RAND Health Program and was funded by the Community Voices–Miami project. Additional support for production of this report was provided by RAND Health. The report should be useful to those in the health care community in Miami-Dade County, as well as to others interested in the issue of governance for public health policy and delivery.

---

[1] United Way of Miami-Dade was asked to join the effort to provide assistance with community outreach.

Contents

Figures

Summary

In Miami-Dade County, Florida, health care for the medically uninsured is provided primarily by the county-run system, the Public Health Trust (PHT), which operates a number of facilities, including the prestigious Jackson Memorial Hospital (JMH) and a network of primary-care clinics. This centralized system has led to uninsured patients having less-convenient access to publicly funded inpatient care than insured county residents have.

When the PHT was first created by the Miami-Dade Board of County Commissioners (BCC) in 1973, there was a transparent reporting mechanism that provided the county with important oversight into how public funds were spent. Hospital management submitted detailed billing statements to county management for all indigent-care patients treated at JMH. While the county often did not reimburse the hospital fully for the care provided, there was clear accounting for indigent care provided and the public dollars used to pay for that care.

In addition to monitoring accountability of public funds, the BCC was actively involved in the selection of PHT board members. The Health Systems Agency (HSA) (which no longer exists) would identify three nominees for each vacancy, and the BCC made the final selection.

Funding for the PHT changed in 1991, when the county passed a special half-penny surtax to provide funds to support JMH. These funds were earmarked "for the operation, maintenance and administration of Jackson Memorial Hospital to improve health care services."[1] The infusion of funds financially stabilized the institution, but it broke the clear accountability and reporting mechanism, since the surtax revenues were treated like a block grant. The surtax funds also provided an opportunity for the BCC to move other health-related programs into the PHT budget, giving the PHT significant oversight of health care for the entire county.

In addition to operating the public health care facilities in Miami-Dade County, the PHT is charged by ordinance to develop and implement plans for the countywide provision of health care services to the uninsured. This dual mission

---

[1] Language on the referendum ballot.

of service provision and countywide planning inherently creates a conflict of interest. That is, the best governance structure for an organization that operates the health care facilities may not be the best governance structure for the organization responsible for countywide health care policy planning. This conflict of interest potentially prevents the organization from performing either function well.

Over the years, the loss of the reporting mechanism and the resulting apparent lack of transparency and accountability have disturbed many county residents. In response to this and other public concerns, the current mayor of Miami-Dade County, Alex Penelas, convened a health care task force in February 2002 charged with, among other tasks, examining the governance, planning, and organization of the publicly funded health care programs in the county.

As a partner in the Community Voices–Miami project, RAND was asked by the project's oversight team and leadership to examine the issues concerning governance. Specifically, RAND researchers were asked to synthesize the literature on governance, to examine how other localities provide health care for the uninsured, and to relate their findings to the publicly funded health care system in Miami-Dade County.

This report discusses the principles of good governance as outlined by Carver (2002) and Pointer and Orlikoff (1999, 2002a,b) in their writings on nonprofit organizational governance. These principles highlight the primary role of the public (or "owners") in governing a public enterprise and the importance of separating the board from management. To reinforce this separateness, the governing body must address two key questions: For whom are we governing? For what are we governing? The answers to these questions naturally lead the governing body to consider policies that can enable management to attain the organization's mission.

The policy governance paradigm emphasizes policy development rather than management skills (Carver, 2002). Importantly, it also emphasizes independence of action—the board does more than just rubber-stamp management's plans and actions. Pointer and Orlikoff (2002a) identified 64 principles of policy governance, which we used as a guide for the study reported here. These principles stress having a board that is committed and impartial, actively overseeing the operations of the organization. Two principles address the board's overall role and its relationship with management:

- The board realizes that it alone bears ultimate responsibility, authority, and accountability for the organization. It understands the importance of governance and undertakes its work with a sense of seriousness and purpose (Principle 1).[2]

- The board does not become directly involved in developing organizational strategies; it delegates this task to management (Principle 12).

We examine how these principles mirror those outlined in the PHT bylaws. Much of the structure required for good governance is stipulated there. However, we identified two broad issues that violate the principles of policy governance: First, as noted above, the PHT both operates its own facilities, which provide considerable uncompensated care, and is responsible for countywide planning for the provision of health care services to the uninsured. Second, the level of accountability among the PHT, the BCC, and county residents has eroded, reducing public trust.

In addition to these two broad issues, there are lapses in the execution of good governance principles that ultimately affect the PHT's accountability and transparency as a public organization.

Areas in Which Governance Needs Improvement

Board and CEO Relations

Several principles for good governance apply specifically to the relationship between the board and the chief executive officer (CEO). As a direct report to the board, the CEO is accountable to the board, and the board is responsible for evaluating his or her performance. Specifically, according to the principles of good governance,

- The board has a CEO succession plan (Principle 16).
- Annually, employing explicit criteria, the board assesses the CEO's performance and contributions (Principle 18).
- Annually, the board adjusts the CEO's compensation (Principle 19).

In one recent and very public example, the board asked the president and CEO of the PHT to resign. (And he did.) The PHT had not evaluated his performance for the previous five years and had not reviewed his compensation, nor had it developed a succession plan. Several months later, the board turned around and

---

[2]The 64 principles are reproduced in the Appendix to this report.

removed the board chairman, who had initiated the CEO's resignation, arguably questioning board decisions made in the prior months.

Board Composition

The PHT could also improve its composition, in accordance with two relevant principles:

- Board composition is nonrepresentational (Principle 53).
- Insiders and those servicing *ex officio* comprise less than 25 percent of the board's membership (Principle 55).

The PHT board has 21 voting and 8 *ex officio* members who are its own employees and employees of the University of Miami. The 21 include a representative of the University of Miami, a private institution that operates the medical school and staffs the PHT facilities. There is a clear potential for conflict of interest, and this situation has endured for many years.

Regular Assessment of the Governance Structure

The mayor's task force has motivated the community generally, and the PHT specifically, in line with the principle that

- Governance structure is thoroughly assessed at regular intervals and modified if necessary (Principle 46).

Specific Recommendations

A good governance structure attempts to relate the organization's mission to its activities, reduce the opportunity for board involvement in management activities, eliminate potential conflicts of interest, and provide a clear accountability of services provided to the indigent and public funds expended. In our investigation of ways to improve the governance of Miami-Dade County publicly funded health care, we assessed how other localities have provided care for their uninsured and underinsured residents. For example, the Health Care District (HCD) of Palm Beach County contracts with private providers who, in turn, treat uninsured persons. The HCD board has access to all information about service provision and can make this publicly available. Another locality, St. Louis, Missouri, provides explicit opportunities for community input on how and what services are provided. Finally, Johns Hopkins Medicine uses well-structured, decentralized governance boards for a complex academic medical center and affiliated institutions.

Using the principles of good governance as the framework, along with the lessons learned from other locales, we make the recommendations outlined below.

Separate the Provision of Services from Planning

Our examination of the PHT's organizational mission—the provision of services and the planning for the health care needs of Miami-Dade County residents—reveals an inherent conflict of interest. Because the PHT board is responsible for the operations and viability of the various Jackson Health System facilities, its prime concern is with that system. However, as a major policy and planning body for the county, the PHT is ultimately accountable to the county for assuring that public funds are allocated appropriately to assure that adequate health care services are available to the uninsured.

To eliminate this potential conflict between services provision and planning and policy, we recommend that the Miami-Dade County BCC separate these two functions. Fortunately, legislative language is already in place that allows for this separation to be implemented. We recommend that the PHT be renamed the Board of Trustees for the Jackson Health System (BTJHS) and that it govern the network of facilities that comprise that system. We recommend that the PHT's countywide planning function be completely turned over to the Health Policy Authority (or some similar entity), which could be renamed the Health Policy Trust (HPT) to reflect its new role as an independent body. We additionally recommend that the BCC consolidate other health care policy and planning activities and their related funding into the HPT. The intent is to transfer indigent-health-care planning duties from all entities under the purview of the county and empower the new HPT to perform those functions. Implementing these recommendations would realign the missions of these two distinct bodies and would eliminate the inherent conflict of interest.

We recommend that in the process of separating these functions, the structure and composition of the boards should be carefully reviewed and revised. In particular, the size and composition of the boards could be modified to improve governance, and better reporting of board activities would enhance accountability and transparency.

Provide Adequate Funding for Planning and Charity Care

The HPT will require adequate funding to carry out its newly consolidated planning and policy activities. Various funding strategies should be considered by the BCC, including diverting extant public funds from other programs, raising additional or new taxes, and allowing the HPT to obtain grant and contract funding. Building a diverse funding base for health to the uninsured and underinsured would provide needed stability for patients as well as providers.

For an example of how extant public funds could be diverted to the HPT, we examined the funding approach that the PHT considered in response to the Lacasa Bill (HB71, 2000).[3] The compromise language approved by the PHT in this resolution provided for incremental funding to a new, independent health authority that would then reimburse community providers for health care to the indigent. Specifically, the PHT resolution proposed that this new authority receive (from PHT funds) $10 million in year 1, $15 million in year 2, and $21.9 million in years 3 through 5.[4] Miami-Dade County was to provide matching funds, resulting in over $180 million of public funds being diverted to the new independent health authority in the first five years. If the BCC were to follow this funding allocation formula for the HPT (or a similar entity), this new body would have the resources necessary to carry out the planning and evaluation of countywide health care, as well as to implement new mechanisms to directly fund care for the uninsured.

In addition to reallocating existing tax funding, the BCC could consider additional tax-based strategies. Raising taxes in the current economic and political climate may seem difficult, but other localities have had success when taxes are targeted to specific programs that the public feels are necessary. Finally, the HPT should be given the authority to secure grant and contract funding (such authority is not explicitly included in the HPT ordinance language), since private foundations and federal agencies fund much innovation in the health care arena. Moreover, the HPT should become a leader in innovation regarding expansions of Medicaid and other federal-state programs.

---

[3]This amendment proposed diverting up to 25 percent of the county's maintenance-of-effort (MOE) funds currently allocated to the PHT to a special fund to be administered by a board independent from that which runs the county public hospital, to provide some level of reimbursement to all eligible hospitals within the county that provide health care services to the indigent. This amendment would transform the Miami-Dade County system into one in which, at least to some degree, dollars follow the patient. Although the bill was passed by the Florida State Legislature, it ultimately was found to violate Miami-Dade County's Home Rule Law and was found to be unconstitutional.

[4]Resolution PHT 04/00-051, described in the PHT minutes for April 26, 2000.

Conclusions

Because the PHT leadership is currently in transition, it is an opportune time to make changes. This opportunity was succinctly summarized by the mayor when he wrote to the PHT:

> Moreover, it is critical that the responsibilities of the new President be clearly defined. Whether the new President will be in charge of the County's entire health care system or of operating Jackson Memorial Hospital, or both, is a basic policy issue. These are among the prevailing health care issues currently being discussed by the members of Mayor's Health Care Access Task Force. The timing for this community debate could not be more appropriate but it must occur before the search process comes to a conclusion. (Penelas, 2002)

Thus, Miami-Dade County is poised on the threshold of decision. It can continue doing business as before, tolerating the dual mission of the PHT and the potential conflicts of interest, or it can move ahead and transform its institutions to better serve its community. It is up to the community and its elected officials to designate a governance structure that allows for inclusive and transparent policymaking concerning Miami-Dade's medically uninsured.

Acknowledgments

The authors wish to thank all those who contributed directly and indirectly to this study. In particular, we thank the many people in Miami-Dade County who have been open and forthcoming with us during the five years we studied the policy processes that address access to health care for the medically uninsured. We wish to thank the members of the Community Voices–Miami project team, including Leda Pérez, Elise Linder, Heather Harrison, and Claudia Hernandez, for their support. We thank Hilary Hoo-you and Marty Lucia of the Miami-Dade County Health Policy Authority, who reviewed much of Chapter 5 and provided additional information and suggestions to assure factual accuracy of the material included therein. We also thank Tanya Palmer of the Health Care District of Palm Beach County and Robert Fruend of the St. Louis Regional Health Commission for providing information about their public health care systems.

We additionally would like to thank our reviewers, John W. Colloton, Director Emeritus, University of Iowa Hospitals and Clinics, and Donna Farley, RAND Senior Health Policy Scientist. The report also benefited from the comments of James Chiesa of RAND. Finally, we would like to thank Louis Ramirez for his assistance in preparing the final document.

Any errors are, of course, the responsibility of the authors.

Acronyms and Abbreviations

BCC	Miami-Dade Board of County Commissioners
BTJHS	Board of Trustees, Jackson Health System (proposed)
CalPERS	California Public Employees' Retirement System
CBO	Community-based organization
CCP	Coordinated Care Program
CEO	Chief executive officer
CVM	Community Voices—Miami
DSH	Disproportionate share hospital
DSS	State of Missouri, Department of Social Services
HCD	Health Care District of Palm Beach County
HCGH	Howard County General Hospital
HPA	Health Policy Authority of Miami-Dade County
HPT	Health Policy Trust (proposed)
HSA	Health Systems Agency
JHBMC	Johns Hopkins Bayview Medical Center
JHH	Johns Hopkins Hospital
JHHCS	Johns Hopkins Health Care System
JHM	Johns Hopkins Medicine
JMH	Jackson Memorial Hospital
JSCH	Jackson South Community Hospital
MOE	Maintenance of effort
OIG	Office of the Inspector General
PHT	Public Health Trust
RDFA	St. Louis Regional Disproportionate Share Hospital Funding Authority
RHC	St. Louis Regional Health Commission
TIAA-CREF	Teachers Insurance and Annuity Association–College Retirement Equities Fund

1. Introduction

More than 40 million Americans were without health insurance in 2001, and the number is expected to grow (Agency for Healthcare Research and Quality, 2002). The economic slump following September 11, 2001, caused some employers to reduce employee benefits or increase cost-sharing in employer-sponsored health insurance policies. In addition, tax revenues used to pay for public health care programs, such as Medicaid, are declining, making it that much more difficult for individuals without health insurance to obtain access to health care services (Hebert, 2002).

Concern for the uninsured is not new, and the number of proposals for effectively providing better health care access for all is increasing. In 1998, the W. K. Kellogg Foundation launched a five-year initiative, Community Voices, in response to concerns about access to health care by the uninsured. The initiative funded 13 sites nationally to assist local organizations in strengthening community support services, giving the underserved a voice in the debate over health care access, and identifying ways to meet the needs of the uninsured and underinsured. One of the Community Voices grants went to Camillus House, a Catholic social service agency and health care provider for the homeless in Miami. RAND was asked to evaluate the Community Voices–Miami (CVM) project and provide technical assistance.

CVM requested that RAND conduct a study of the governance structure of the Miami-Dade County Public Health Trust (PHT) to help the project's oversight team and staff better understand issues related to governance, and to provide them with information for participating in local policy discussions. This report reviews the principles of good governance, provides examples of governance structures used by other health organizations, compares and contrasts the principles with the structure and function of the PHT, and offers recommendations for improvement.

This study continues RAND's participation in the CVM effort, providing technical assistance and analysis of the public provision of health care services to the uninsured of Miami-Dade County. The first technical assistance report for this project, *Hospital Care for the Uninsured in Miami-Dade County: Hospital Finance and Patient Travel Patterns* (Jackson et al., 2002), examined aggregate hospital financing and revenue flows and patient travel patterns to the county's 24 acute-care hospitals. It found that, among the county's providers of health care to the indigent, Jackson Memorial Hospital (JMH), Miami-Dade County's public hospital run by the PHT, provides the vast majority of charity care. Although there are private hospitals closer to their homes, uninsured patients living in remote areas of the county travel to JMH for care. Similar travel patterns were not seen among patients who had health insurance. The report concluded that centralization of funding for and the location of the county's public hospital facilities have created disparities in geographic access between uninsured and insured patients.

Concern about providing health care services to the uninsured has been further elevated by concern about governance in Miami-Dade County. In this report, we examine governance generally and consider governance of the PHT specifically as it relates to its responsibility for the health of county residents. The PHT currently comprises numerous facilities, including JMH, which is staffed by University of Miami physicians. The PHT, with an annual operating budget of more than $1 billion, has one board that not only governs PHT facilities but also is expected to consider countywide health care policy. There are more than 20 private not-for-profit and for-profit hospitals in the county, two of which are public and under the authority of the PHT. The PHT board generally focuses on its own network of facilities, rather than working closely with other providers who may be able to provide services to the uninsured that are less costly or more geographically accessible.

On February 15, 2002, Miami-Dade County Mayor Alex Penelas launched a task force to look into issues of the uninsured, including governance and how the county spends its funds on health care for the indigent. Several months later, PHT Chairman Michael Kosnitzky established an ad hoc subcommittee to examine the governance of the PHT. It is within this environment of concern that we undertook this study of governance. We have abstracted from the literature those concepts, structures, and processes that can facilitate good governance. Our conclusions are based on the fundamental belief that although organizations differ in their goals and means, there are certain principles that all organizations must consider when designing or redesigning their governance bodies.

In this report, we first define governance and describe why governance is an important issue for public health care. We then set out principles of governance that should be considered by any governing body. These principles not only provide a structure for good governance, they also direct boards to actively govern. This combination of structure and action makes good governance feasible. We illustrate these principles through several examples of organizational governance for public and private entities that provide health care services. We then turn to the specific system of public health care in Miami-Dade County and compare the principles of good governance with the PHT ordinance, bylaws, and activities. Finally, we present some recommendations and consider the policy implications of those recommendations.

2. What Is Governance? Why Is It Needed?

Governance is defined as the exercise of authority and a method or system of government or management (*Webster's Unabridged Dictionary*, 1997). Issues of governance concern all organizations, from large for-profit corporations to governmental agencies to small nonprofit community-based organizations (CBOs). In particular, we are concerned with the governance of nonprofit organizations and governmental agencies involved in health care.

Governance often is performed by a board that provides oversight and ensures accountability of an organization to its owners and stakeholders. The governing board is ultimately responsible for the success of the organization. This chapter examines the way governing boards conduct their business.

Much of the literature on governance relates specifically to publicly traded corporations, where the focus is on accountability, responsibility, and profitability. Today, corporate governance and the methods used by corporate boards to monitor corporate activities have taken on greater significance than they had in previous times. Future history books may label the turn of the 21st century as a period of corporate corruption and mistrust in America. The spectacular financial disasters of companies such as Enron, Arthur Andersen, WorldCom, and Tyco sensitized the public to variations and excesses in accounting practices. Transparency and accountability have thus become valued practices, and the public is more alert than ever to the potential for conflicts of interest. There is a general concern that many boards are not providing the requisite level of oversight and are failing to rein in management. While regulatory means have yet to be established to prevent future debacles, the public has called for change in the way business is done.

These concerns, however, are not focused solely on corporate America. Distrust of government and nonprofit agencies has also grown. As far back as 1978, the year in which California's Proposition 13 passed,[1] taxpayers were beginning to ask whether the government was doing the right thing with their money. Polls show that this continues to be a concern (Roper Center, 2002), and it might be posited that bond or other funding issues have failed in part because of voters'

---

[1]Proposition 13 was a tax-reform initiative proposed by Howard Jarvis that cut property taxes by 30 percent and capped annual increases (Moore, 1998).

perception of a lack of accountability and transparency in government funding and allocation decisions. In the nonprofit sector, donors have come to rely on the reports of services that rate charities (e.g., based on the proportion of contributions that actually goes to "people in need" versus administration), and accounting practices at well-respected organizations such as United Way are coming under increasing scrutiny (Strom, 2002).

Governance is not a new concept, but there has been a recent shift in thinking about what constitutes good governance. This new paradigm, policy governance, was initially described by Carver and Carver (2001) and was elaborated on in Carver (2002). It was further refined and articulated by Pointer and Orlikoff (1999, 2002a,b), among others. Their work forms the basis of much of Chapter 3 of this report, in which we discuss the specific principles illustrated by the concept. Other authors have written on issues similar or complementary to governance, and, where possible, these are also included in the discussion.

Policy governance, as proposed by Carver, is a theory of governing the public's business, i.e., how governance connects the "public" to public enterprise (Carver, 2002). As such, governance derives not from management, but from ownership (Carver, 2002). Governing boards take the interests and needs of owners and stakeholders and meld them into organizational objectives that are executed by management. Carver's model builds upon previous work, in particular, social contract philosophy, Greenleaf's concept of servant-leadership (see, for example, Greenleaf, 1977), and modern management. However, the policy governance model highlights the primary role of the public (or "owners") in governing the public enterprise and the separateness of the board from management. As Carver explains:

> Rather than a theory of execution, it is a theory of ownership and the expression of ownership in the organizational context. It positions the board as a completely separate function facing the ownership in the primary direction and the executive organization [management] in the other—quite different from seeing governance as an extension or subdiscipline of management. It requires board members to be servant-leaders rather than either demagogues or administrators. (Carver, 2002, p. 10)

The policy governance paradigm emphasizes policy development, rather than management skills. Importantly, it also emphasizes action—good governance is not mere rubber-stamping of management's plans and actions. Modern policy formulation and monitoring require a set of interpersonal communication skills to bring multiple stakeholders together in a constructive, productive, and mutually respectful way. Salamon (2001) calls these interpersonal communication skills "enablement skills"—activation, orchestration, and modulation skills—to highlight the importance of moving from the traditional directive approach of governance to the more cooperative or interdependent mode of action that policy formulation requires. For example, to incorporate stakeholder perspectives into the policy discussion, it is necessary to activate owner and stakeholder community networks to identify problems and develop solutions. The board's role is to coordinate all input from these networks and act as the "orchestra conductor." In orchestrating activities and input, the board must be able to synthesize ideas, identify themes, and develop policies accordingly. Finally, in setting policy, the board must be able to anticipate the consequences of its actions and balance gains and losses within the context of the mission of the organization and its place in the community.

Convening concerned stakeholders and developing networks of nonprofit or governmental agencies take time and bring the risk of losing discretion over the use of public authority and the spending of public funds (Salamon, 2001). As more individuals and agencies get involved in solving public problems, centralized control may appear to dissipate. For example, when public agencies contract out for services, monitoring, which was previously an agency function, becomes part of the contracting processes. Agencies are challenged to define measures that permit monitoring of the quality of the services provided. Privatization moves monitoring even further away from direct governmental control. While efficiency motives often drive the move to privatization, efficiency may come at the expense of transparency, integrity, and accountability (Schooner, 2001). To avoid these problems, governance principles and actions need to be updated. As noted by Schooner, "If government plans to follow a private sector model, its greatest chance of success in serving the public while maintaining the public's trust would be to integrate a robust public oversight regime into that model" (Schooner, 2001).

Interestingly, much of the rhetoric about policy governance is consistent with the rhetoric about accountability in general. While the focus is slightly different, the discussion about accountability of resources, outcomes, and processes is complementary to that of policy governance (Kearns, 1996).

Good governance not only requires fastidious attention to legal and regulatory details, it also entails a cognizance of owner and stakeholder perceptions and trust. Even when certain checks and balances are in place to reveal objective evidence of poor governance and trigger remedial action, perceptions of poor governance can destroy the trust that many organizations rely on to conduct their business. Over the past decade, two large nonprofit retirement plans, California Public Employees' Retirement System (CalPERS) and Teachers Insurance and Annuity Association–College Retirement Equities Fund (TIAA-

CREF),[2] have developed criteria for good governance and, when appropriate, have demanded that companies in which they invest improve their governance. With their significant financial investment, CalPERS and TIAA-CREF have had considerable leverage over corporate boards. More recently, on a smaller but still significant scale, a major private donor in Cleveland withheld donations because he was displeased with the governance of various public institutions in the city. His frustration as a donor-stakeholder was ignited when the costs of a university building to which he had donated escalated. He held the university board responsible for not appropriately monitoring the building costs and withheld his philanthropic giving until changes were made in the various governing boards (Winter, 2002).

Nowhere is trust among stakeholders more important than in the health care field today. Public and private health care organizations are faced with increasing costs, decreasing reimbursement levels, and increasing numbers of uninsured persons in their communities. Many struggle to stay afloat, while others implement aggressive pricing "strategies" to game the system. Some even blame the huge increases in the cost of medical care on these strategies, which, though often legal, can lead to mistrust among stakeholders (*Los Angeles Times*, 2002).

Trust can facilitate collaboration among stakeholders (health care systems, providers, community organizations), and collaboration is important because rarely can a single organization improve community health *by itself* (Annison and Wilford, 1998). The challenges facing the health care sector are too great for any one organization and often require multisector approaches. Why, then, does effective collaboration not always occur? Annison and Wilford (1998) identify two barriers: "the curse of success," and ego and institutional pride. Successful organizations are often accustomed to operating independently—they may not have developed trusting relationships with others and may have a hard time seeing why they *need* to collaborate. Institutional pride leads board members to focus on the health system, bottom line, or competition, at the expense of community needs. Both of these barriers to collaboration can be overcome with good governance.

It is important to recognize that although governance relates to management, it is not the same as management. Management should focus on the day-to-day operation of an organization, while the governing board is responsible for establishing the mission, objectives, and program policy under which

---

[2]For more information on these plans, see http://www.calpers-governance.org and http://www.tiaa-cref.org/pubs/pdf/InvestPhilosophy.pdf.

management operates. Boards develop the policy structure—the "Thou shalls" and "Thou shall nots"—i.e., the rules by which management operates. The board should not micromanage operations. For some boards, this is a radical shift. In discussing the need for overhaul of many hospital boards, Carver noted:

> The intention of this radical shift in the rules of governance is that management be allowed as much room to move as is prudent and ethical, so long as managers understand that the real reason for the organization to exist is not survival itself or organizational size and prestige. The reason is that human beings in need are better off, that lives are improved, that pain is lessened, that the unhappy effects of trauma and disease are minimal. (Carver, 2002, p. 594)

Pressure to improve the governance structure of publicly funded health care in Miami-Dade County is motivated by the desire to increase access to care for the near half-million uninsured people in the county. Good governance will engender trust, and trust will facilitate collaboration among providers in the community to improve the health and health care access of residents. A board that discharges its duties responsibly, with transparency and accountability, will also engender these same qualities in others (McDonough, 2002).

3. A Primer on Governance

In this chapter, we discuss governance, both conceptually and practically. Because we are interested in the governance of public funds and programs, we focus on nonprofit organizations and governmental agencies where boards of directors, trustees, or advisors[1] are involved in organizational oversight. Our discussion is enriched by the discourse in the for-profit sector, where many of the principles of governance have recently been reexamined and rearticulated. These corporate principles are helpful in the Miami-Dade context; indeed, many of the principles of good governance apply to organizations of all types. The PHT, clearly a governmental agency, was established by county ordinance in 1973, specifically giving the board of trustees "the powers, duties and responsibilities customarily vested in the board of directors of a private corporation."[2] Thus, this primer reflects a synthesis of the literature and practice of governance from both the for-profit and nonprofit sectors.

The policy governance conceptual model developed by Carver and Carver (2001) is applicable to various organizations, including nonprofits. It articulates a new board-management relationship and assigns to the board the responsibility for policy development and assessment. By moving away from the minutiae of operations statistics and focusing on the larger issues of organizational mission, vision, and policy, governing boards can maintain their legal responsibilities while facilitating organizational development and growth. A board that articulates its organization's mission and policies clearly also establishes benchmarks with which to assess organizational and chief executive officer (CEO) performance.

Two features of policy governance provide an overarching vision for board governance: (1) development and promulgation of clear objectives for the board (its chair and its members), the CEO, and the organization, and (2) assessment of performance—of the organization, the CEO, and board members—based on these clear objectives and, as required, board decisionmaking and action. Good governance requires that when deficiencies are identified, the board be willing to take action, such as removing the CEO or requesting more frequent reporting of pertinent performance measures. Many boards have traditionally focused on

---

[1]We will henceforth use the terms *board* and *board member*.
[2]Miami-Dade County Ordinance 73-69.

past performance and rubber-stamped management decisions, but it is the continuous process of statement, assessment, reflection, and retooling that defines policy governance. It focuses discussion and activity on improvement and prepares the organization to meet the challenges that lie ahead.

In the discussion below, we refer to 64 principles of governance defined by Pointer and Orlikoff (2002a).[3] These principles are consistent with other work on governance and provide a simple catalog of concepts and activities that any board should consider. The first two principles relate to the tone and commitment with which a board functions rather than to specific actions. Principle 1 states:

> The board realizes that it alone bears ultimate responsibility, authority, and accountability for the organization. It understands the importance of governance and undertakes its work with a sense of seriousness and purpose.

Similarly, Principle 2 states that the board understands those factors that affect good governance and therefore adheres to a set of principles under which it governs. To further emphasize the importance of the board's attitude, Pointer and Orlikoff (2002a) add two other principles: the board develops policies addressing its ultimate responsibilities, and it makes the decisions that are required of it.[4] Thus, boards can have the structure for good governance (that is, appropriate bylaws, mission statements, etc.), but without a sense of responsibility and resolve to set policy and act as necessary, they cannot effect good governance. The core roles for the board are policy formulation, decisionmaking and action, and oversight.[5]

As should be clear, Pointer and Orlikoff (2002a) distinguish their ideas of boards and governance from the perhaps more historical conceptualizations of nonprofit organization boards as being primarily interested in fundraising and social status rather than in true governance. This report also views governance as the exercise of authority or method of government or management.

The Board's Role and Responsibilities

The most important discussion a board should undertake is centered on two questions: For whom are we governing? For what are we governing?

---

[3]These principles are reproduced in the Appendix to this report. In subsequent work, Pointer and Orlikoff (2002b) have expanded the number of principles to 72. Some of these recent additions are incorporated into the discussion.

[4]Principles 32 and 33.

[5]Principle 31.

Governance for Whom? Boards represent owners. In the nonprofit arena, they have also come to represent stakeholder perspectives. All owners are stakeholders, but not all stakeholders are owners.[6] It is important that the board understand the difference. Boards must balance stakeholders' interests within the constraints of the organization's mission and viability. The board translates owner interests into strategic policy and action (Carver, 2002). Thus, one of the most important tasks of a board is to identify the organization's owners and stakeholders.[7]

Many nonprofit organizations are established to provide services to particular subpopulations defined by characteristics such as neighborhood or residence, demographics, etc. For example, an organization may be established to provide services solely to the elderly or to persons with HIV. Other organizations may have more diverse sets of stakeholders, making the identification of owners and stakeholders elusive. Community hospitals, for example, often have as their mission the provision of services to the community, neighborhood, or catchment area in which they are located. However, a particular hospital may be owned by a religious organization, a nonprofit organization, or a for-profit organization. Board members must know for whom they are working when they deliberate and make policy decisions for an organization. Thus, one might expect different hospital boards to develop different policies and make different decisions.

It is common for nonprofit boards to have members who reflect subgroups of owners and stakeholders. Board members, however, should not act as constituent representatives. They serve as owner-agents and ultimately must balance their views and interests with those of the organization.[8] This role is important to consider when developing procedures for board membership nomination. While there may be a desire to have the composition of the board reflect different constituencies, board work is not representative government.

Boards can make the mistake of considering management and other staff as owners. Certainly, staff are stakeholders, but they generally are not owners. The direction of authority is from the board to management. That is, management works for the board. The board must thus be prepared to carefully monitor and assess the organization's management.

Governance for What? Nonprofit organizations and governmental agencies often have missions more diffuse than those of for-profit organizations, where

---

[6]The distinction between owners and stakeholders is more relevant in the for-profit sector, where there are equity owners.

[7]Principle 4.

[8]Principle 53.

the objective is profit maximization. Nonprofit organizations often have less-pecuniary missions, such as providing health services to all members of the community regardless of their ability to pay or maintaining and improving the health of the community. Ultimately, however, the board is responsible for the financial viability of the organization. Therefore, boards of nonprofits must be prepared to monitor and assess a broad range of outcomes and products in order to assure that their organizations are carrying out their missions appropriately.

An initial and recurrent task of the board is to articulate the mission of the organization. The mission statement establishes for whom and for what the board governs. The work of the board follows according to a set of governance principles. In the remainder of this chapter, we further examine the board's role and responsibilities.

Board Work

Having identified its owners, stakeholders, and mission, the governing board must focus on policy formulation and develop a further understanding of the owners' and stakeholders' expectations for the organization. Through outreach into the community, the board can learn firsthand stakeholder and owner concerns and the role the organization can play in the community. Such outreach reinforces the need on the part of the board to periodically ask who the owners and stakeholders are and what they expect of the board and the organization.[9] Once these are understood, the board can act on their behalf in discharging its duties.[10]

The board, having ultimate organizational responsibility, must also assure that the organization meets all regulatory requirements within various legal constraints. Policy governance is not an alternative to these legal regulations; rather, it facilitates the board's service to the twin "bosses" of owners and stakeholders and the law.[11]

The approach of policy governance moves the board away from monitoring the minutiae of operations statistics to developing policies and monitoring key metrics reflecting the stated objectives for the organization. Board committees develop measures to assess whether the organization's objectives are being met. Committee work involves determining what needs to be measured and reported

---

[9]Principles 4 and 5.
[10]Principle 6.
[11]Principles 6, 7, and 8.

by management so that the board can fulfill its fiduciary and legal responsibilities.

To assure the organization's success, the board must develop clear plans for meeting clearly stated objectives[12] and must articulate them in clearly written vision statements, policies, and statements of expected outcomes.[13] The CEO and his or her management team can then work within these broad parameters and marshal resources to accomplish the board's organizational goals.[14] Importantly, these written statements form the basis of the CEO's performance evaluation.

The board and its committees should annually set out their objectives for the year.[15] These objectives help keep the board and committee work focused and facilitate scheduling board activities and deliberations.

The board should also measure and monitor the quality of services or products produced by the organization. The organization's reputation and future viability—maintenance of which is the board's primary objective—are based on the quality of its product. Thus, the board must make decisions about what the organization produces, what constitutes high quality, and what makes business sense.[16] The board or its quality committee must develop a set of quality indicators that can be measured and periodically reported on by management.[17] These quality indicators should be defined to reflect organizational practices as well as to reveal problems, so that the board has sufficient information with which to take remedial action or refine organizational policies.[18]

As part of its responsibility for the fiscal viability of the organization, the board must put in place policies that assure that the organization works within stated regulations. The board or the finance committee establishes financial objectives and recommends financial indicators, reported on by management, for use by the board in its monitoring activities. Like the product and quality measures, the financial indicators should follow practice and provide information to enable the board to make decisions if remediation is required.[19] The board is responsible for assuring that the necessary financial controls are in place to satisfy regulators,

---

[12]Principle 9.

[13]Principles 10 and 11.

[14]Principle 12.

[15]Principle 58.

[16]Principles 21 and 22.

[17]Principle 23.

[18]Principle 24.

[19]Principles 25, 26, 27, 28, and 29.

as well as assuring that there is accountability to owners and stakeholders for how funds are spent. Accountability and transparency are achieved through rigorous internal controls, including internal and external audits. In addition to meeting regulatory requirements, the auditing process can reveal practices and procedures that should be updated. The board should be prepared to address such issues through updating polices and procedures.

Ultimately, the board should have a substantial degree of autonomy from management and external influences. The board needs a budget and adequate staff support with which to conduct its work,[20] and, when necessary, it should be able to engage outside experts to assist with governance issues.

A final hallmark of an effectively functioning governing board is its devotion of time to forward strategic thinking, rather than retrospective monitoring.[21] If the board has developed appropriate indices, monitoring should take little time, freeing up the board to consider the future direction of the organization and to anticipate challenges.

The board chair should establish an environment where discussion can be open and honest, without threat of recrimination (Carver, 2002). Healthy discussion is essential—in its absence, board decisions may be made without full information or understanding. However, once a decision has been made, all board members should support it.[22] Division among board members can cripple a board and hinder an organization.

In sum, the board has two primary responsibilities: First, it must set out clear, written expectations for the CEO and the organization and develop policy values under which the organization is to conduct its business. Second, it must evaluate whether or not these expectations have been met, by monitoring meaningful indicators of performance. When clear expectations are set and meaningful indices are monitored, the board must then be prepared to take action if it finds deficiencies.

Board Member Responsibilities

To function appropriately, board members must have explicit performance expectations, education, and training. Performance criteria may be both administrative (e.g., meeting attendance) and functional (e.g., contribution to

---

[20]Principles 56 and 57.
[21]Principles 34 and 35.
[22]Principle 36.

board work). The board is responsible for its performance and contribution to the organization,[23] and its members must be committed to their work and prepared to assess and take action.

Administrative Criteria. The dynamic nature of many sectors of the economy, especially health care, requires that board members be appropriately oriented and that they be offered opportunities for further training and education. New board member training should occur early in a member's tenure in order to maximize his or her participation. Pointer and Orlikoff (2002a) recommend new member training within three months of joining a board,[24] and at least biannual external training for board member development.[25] In addition to meeting regularly, the board should have periodic retreats, the frequency of which depends on the amount of policy work that needs to be done.[26] For boards involved in restructuring and transforming, quarterly retreats may be required (Pointer and Orlikoff, 2002a).

Functional Criteria. To enhance board functioning, members should have written job descriptions that clearly define their roles and responsibilities (McAdam and Gies, 1990),[27] and they should be committed to carrying out their duties.[28] The job description should also explicitly include the length and number of terms that a member may serve[29] and should describe meeting attendance goals beyond simple requirements for a quorum.

Further, board members' performance should be evaluated periodically.[30] Evaluations can be conducted by board members themselves as a self-assessment exercise or can involve a 360 review[31] by the full board. Whatever type of evaluation is conducted, it should be objective, based on the explicit performance criteria outlined in the job description. Moreover, if a 360 review is conducted, the board should provide a mechanism for performance feedback to enable individuals to improve their performance. Evaluations should occur before a member is asked to serve an additional term, and the board should explicitly consider removing nonperforming members.

---

[23]Principle 30.
[24]Principle 49.
[25]Principle 62.
[26]Principle 63.
[27]Principle 50.
[28]Principle 37 and 38.
[29]Principle 51.
[30]Principle 52.

[31]A 360 review involves eliciting performance assessment input from those organizationally above, equal to, and below the reviewee. This contrasts with a traditional performance review, which elicits assessment input from only those persons who supervise or manage the reviewee.

The Board and the CEO

The board-CEO relationship is important because the CEO is the sole organizational officer who reports directly to the board.[32] The board is responsible for the CEO's hiring and the annual setting of organizational goals and expectations. The board is responsible for annually reviewing and setting the CEO's compensation,[33] as well as for developing a CEO succession plan.[34]

Since the board has the ultimate responsibility for the performance of the CEO, it must conduct an annual performance evaluation.[35] It is the board that must remove the CEO, should that be necessary.[36] The board states its expectations for the organization, for the population(s) benefiting from the organization, and the acceptable costs leading to those services, products, or results (Carver, 2002). It also sets the boundaries of acceptable organizational practice. Assessment ultimately comes from monitoring appropriately defined performance indices that reflect both the expectations and the business practice limitations set by the board.

CEO performance evaluation is often conducted by the executive committee. However, it may be preferable to have a committee solely responsible for this function (Pointer and Orlikoff, 2002a). The committee charged with CEO performance assessment should assist the board in establishing clear, written objectives for the CEO and the organization. The board should secure the "buy-in" of the CEO to these objectives via his or her participation in their formulation. Some objectives may be time-sensitive—that is, they may have associated deadlines—while others may be continuous. The objectives must be stated in a manner that guides the CEO and the organization's activities. With written expectations, performance assessment is focused on the issues, rather than on personality or personal style. The board and committee should reconsider and rewrite the performance objectives if there is ambiguity in the assessment criteria. Unambiguously stated objectives assist the CEO in his or her activities and also permit fair performance evaluations.

Many organizations face the issue of whether the chairman/chairwoman of the board should also hold the CEO position. Carver (2002) posits that having the CEO as chairman or a voting member of the board creates potential conflict

---

[32]Principle 14.

[33]Principle 19.

[34]Principle 16.

[35]Principles 13 and 18.

[36]Principles 15, 17, and 20.

because there is no longer a clear distinction between the board and management. However, numerous corporate organizations have CEO board chairmen/chairwomen. To maintain the board-management relationship, CalPERS recommends that the board meet periodically without the CEO and other nonindependent directors. CalPERS further recommends that when the CEO is also the board chairman, a "lead" director should be selected who can facilitate discussion among the independent directors.

Board Structure

The composition of the board's membership should be reviewed periodically and updated to meet the needs of the organization.[37] Ideally, new members should be selected through explicit selection criteria to maintain diversity and requisite skills.[38] Pointer and Orlikoff (2002a) offer a tool to use when profiling current and prospective board members—a matrix of skills, experience, and diversity parameters.

Size. Because the board provides guidance for an organization, board structure and composition are important foundations. If the board is to actively discuss issues and reach consensus, it must be of a manageable size. A board that is too small may suffer from a paucity of points of view or from the dominance of a few; a board that is too large may be intimidating and may reduce active participation in discussion or be too unwieldy to reach consensus (Carver, 2002). There is no ideal number of members for a board. Recommendations vary, but most suggest that a board should have no fewer than nine and no more than 19 members.[39] An odd number of members is recommended to avoid deadlocks.

Composition. Because the board is focused on policy formulation and not on operations, it is important that its members have diverse experiences and skills. This diversity contributes to the board's ability to be well informed and to conduct careful deliberations. The range of skills and experience of members should be appropriate to the work of the board.

The organization's operational perspective is usually provided by *ex officio* members, that is, persons on the board by virtue of the position they hold (Pointer and Orlikoff, 1999). Pointer and Orlikoff (2002a) recommend that the number of *ex officio* members on a board be limited to two or fewer, or that

---

[37]Principle 47.
[38]Principle 48.
[39]Principle 40.

"inside" and *ex officio* members constitute no more than 25 percent of the board.[40] The CEO is generally on the board as a voting *ex officio* member[41] and may in fact constitute the entire insider and *ex officio* contingent of the board. Because *ex officio* members do not have the same term limitations as other board members, their influence can be of long duration, and as a result, *ex officio* members can (inadvertently) influence the board/management relationship. In health care organizations, the physician chief of the medical staff may also hold an *ex officio* position.

Another challenge to board composition occurs when members are also customers of the organization. In specifying the organization's mission, the board implicitly or explicitly defines its customers. Patients are clearly customers of health care organizations, but physicians are also customers in that they can choose whether or not to practice at a particular hospital. Customer needs and interests may be based on individual characteristics or experiences and can be at variance with those of owners, who are focused on aggregate or macro concerns. Another important challenge when customers are on the board is that they can directly access organizational management, while other board members must obey the management chain of command. The clear board-management structure defined by policy governance precludes board members from intruding on management operational prerogatives. Thus, if customers are on the board, it is important to define clearly board member roles and responsibilities. All board members must be committed to the organization and must make decisions based on the best interests of all owners and stakeholders.

Most health care organizations have board members who are physicians, since physicians understand the workings of a hospital or health care facility. *Ex officio* board members may also be physicians. Non-insider physicians, however, can provide needed experience and perspective without posing the potential problem of the physician-customer. Physician or other expert board members should be screened and evaluated through the same process as other board member nominees.

Board composition may be dictated by external regulation, and members may be elected or appointed. Whatever process is used, it is important to guard against constituency-specific dedicated positions. Board members are not representatives of particular viewpoints; rather, they represent all stakeholders and must balance stakeholder interests with those of the organization.[42] Again,

---

[40]Principle 55.

[41]Principle 54.

[42]Principle 53.

it is important to provide adequate orientation and training so that board members can contribute appropriately and effectively.

Conflict of Interest

No matter how carefully board members are selected, conflict-of-interest issues will sometimes arise. When a board member will benefit, either personally or through his or her business, from a board decision, that member should recuse himself or herself from the discussion and the voting.

Often, however, conflicts of interest are more subtle. Board members may be on other organizations' boards. A conflict of interest can occur when a board member is faced with making decisions for one organization that may affect, either positively or negatively, another organization with which he or she is affiliated. This type of conflict of interest can occur, for example, when organizations compete for funding sources. At a minimum, such "interested" board members should recuse themselves, but more effectively, the board should not have members with such potential conflicts.

Recusing oneself from particular discussions or voting eliminates the gross appearance of conflict of interest. However, more subtle forms can exist, especially if board members have strong personal or business relationships among themselves. Such potential conflicts of interest can stifle discussion or generate *quid pro quo* agreements that hinder the board from making well-informed decisions.

Board Officers

The selection of the board chairman is very important,[43] since the chairman sets the tone of board meetings and provides overall leadership. The chairman's interpersonal and communication skills can determine whether the board environment is conducive to frank discussion. Nominations for the chairmanship are usually made by a special committee composed of the current chairman, the CEO, an at-large board member, and a past chairman who is no longer a member of the board. In making their nominations, the committee should review all possible candidates against the skill and experience criteria for the position and the needs of the board vis-à-vis upcoming issues. The tenure of the chair is usually for one year; however, a two-year tenure may be more effective in that it provides time for the chair to influence the board and the

---

[43]Principle 61.

organization. In some organizations, there is a set succession of the vice chairman to the chairmanship. Such fixed selection criteria make it impossible for the board to match current needs with candidates.

Board Committees

Boards are composed of committees that perform much of the board work. Thus, a board's committee structure should be driven by the board's current needs and should be kept simple.[44] However, in many organizations, the committee structure has ossified over the years, resulting in committees functioning beyond the apparent scope of their labels. Pointer and Orlikoff (1999) recommend that all committees be disbanded annually and reconstituted only if they are needed to conduct the business of the following year. This "zero-based" approach is perhaps too drastic, but it highlights the belief that boards can become bureaucracies of standing bodies that are no longer needed. Boards should periodically reexamine their committee structure to assure that the committees are needed, and all standing committees should have an explicit purpose and clear, written expectations for what they will accomplish.[45] The written guidelines should also specify the roles and responsibilities maintained by the parent board.[46]

That said, several types of committees frequently form the core committee structure for health care organizations: executive committee, finance committee, vision and goals (ends) committee, quality and community health committee, and governance committee (Pointer and Orlikoff, 1999, 2002a). The basic functions of each committee are discussed below.

Executive Committee. Historically, the executive committee has the responsibility for making board-level decisions when it is impossible or not feasible for the full board to meet. However, within the paradigm of policy governance, this committee's authority may be problematic. When the executive committee makes decisions for the board, it is insinuating itself between the board and the CEO, and this can create an awkward dynamic, especially if the CEO-board relationship is not well established or smoothly functioning (Carver, 2002). The board can give the executive committee other tasks, such as providing support to the chair and conducting the CEO performance evaluation, improving governance, and planning the board agenda (Pointer and Orlikoff, 1999, 2002a).

---

[44]Principle 39.
[45]Principles 43 through 46.
[46]Principle 41.

By setting the agenda and anticipating trends and events, the executive committee has a strong influence on the action of the board. The agenda should be constructed to manage the meeting time effectively and efficiently.[47] Board meetings are generally conducted by the chair

Finance Committee. This committee is charged with keeping the organization financially viable. Historically, finance committees are involved in the development, review, and monitoring of the organization's budget. Granted, numerous regulations still require the board to review and approve certain financial activities. However, the trend in policy governance is to have the finance committee establish clear financial policies under which the CEO manages the organization and to base reporting more on organizational objectives than on typical accounting spreadsheets.

The finance committee is also responsible for audit activities, serving as the initial board contact for internal auditing staff. The committee, or a subcommittee, also oversees the external audit and reviews the findings before presentation to the full board. Recent corporate financial crises have motivated many to examine the relationship of the external auditor and the organization and to periodically replace the external auditor to assure that there is no conflict of interest. Conflict of interest here can be bred from familiarity; the use of fresh eyes can enhance the benefits of an audit.

Vision and Goals (Ends) Committee. Historically, this committee was often called the planning committee. Under policy governance, it is responsible for helping the board set the mission, vision, and objectives of the organization and, ultimately, the ends to be attained. The governing board sets up these "ends" policies for the organization, but the exact means used to address them are up to the CEO and his or her management team.

Quality and Community Health Committee. This committee assists the board in developing policies to assess the quality of care delivered by the organization. In this role, this committee is also involved in setting policies and objectives regarding customer satisfaction and community relations.

Governance Committee. This committee assists the board in assessing and improving its governance. It is responsible for planning the annual board retreat, as well as board member development. It is also responsible for assessing the

---

[47]Principles 59 and 60.

performance of the board and preparing comments for the full board to consider and take action on, if required.[48]

Taken together, the board committees focus on specific areas of responsibility and advise the full board. The full board, however, is responsible for all final decisions.

Centralized or Decentralized Governance for Complex Organizations

Governance should be structured to meet the needs of the organization and thus can be either centralized or decentralized. A centralized governance structure is typical of single institution/facility organizations, but it can also be used by organizations with various divisions. Many organizations, including those in health care, have developed into networked or integrated organizations through acquisition or creation of specialty divisions. These specialty divisions have both common and separate missions and hence may require their own oversight boards.

In a decentralized structure, membership of subsidiary organizations' boards may be interlocked—that is, members of the parent board may also be members of subsidiary boards. The parent board communicates to the subsidiary through the subsidiary board; it does not communicate directly to the subsidiary CEO. This discipline in communication between the parent and subsidiary is important, as it preserves the relationship of the subsidiary board to the subsidiary CEO. Direct communication from the parent board to a subsidiary CEO would render the subsidiary board useless and remove its authority over the CEO. Recall that the CEO of a subsidiary is an employee of the subsidiary's board (Carver, 2002).

Because communication between parent and subsidiary occurs at the board level, it is achieved through several mechanisms. The parent board may delegate the communication responsibility to a parent board subcommittee, a parent board member liaison, the parent CEO, or the parent board chairman. In deciding on the best approach for communication between the parent and subsidiary boards, the parent board should consider two issues: First, the person tasked with this responsibility speaks for the parent board and not from his or her individual (or subcommittee) perspective. Second, the parent board must consider how it will hold the subsidiary accountable. Given that the only individual accountable to

---

[48]Principle 64.

the parent board is the parent CEO, an effective communication pathway is created when the parent CEO sits on subsidiary boards. To facilitate the creation of an environment conducive to appropriate action, the parent CEO may be given the authority to appoint subsidiary board members, replace board members, and provide the subsidiary board its charge. This latter role is important for reducing the possibility of creating subsidiary boards that oppose or otherwise thwart the fulfillment of parent board expectations. Thus, the parent CEO is given the means to affect performance, and the parent board can effectively hold the parent CEO responsible for the subsidiary organization's performance.

Summary

The preservation of the board-management relationship is of central importance to policy governance. The CEO reports to the board, and the board is ultimately responsible for the activities and success of the organization. Under policy governance, the board should be forward-looking. Board work, therefore, involves the continuous process of statement, assessment, reflection, and retooling to help the organization succeed and meet future challenges. Board work additionally involves outreach to the stakeholder community to update the board members' understanding of stakeholders' needs and expectations.

4. Examples of Governance Structures for Health Care Services

Because the provision of health care to medically uninsured persons is largely a local responsibility, there is tremendous variation in the way local governmental agencies are structured and governed to meet the needs of the uninsured. In this chapter, we describe three models, two public-sector and one private-sector, that feature transparency, accountability, and local participation—characteristics that support good policy governance. These examples do not represent structures that are immediately replicable in Miami-Dade, but each case provides some feature that is relevant to the Miami-Dade context.

We look at one health care district in South Florida, Palm Beach County, because it is geographically proximate to Miami-Dade, serves a population similar to that of Miami-Dade, raises funds through a dedicated tax for health care services, and operates in the Florida legislative regime. We then turn to St. Louis, which is home to a newly established system for addressing the needs of the uninsured through an innovative governance structure. Finally, we look at a private-sector, multifacility, academic medical center, Johns Hopkins Medicine, which has a well-structured, decentralized board with clearly defined objectives and responsibilities.

Palm Beach County

The Health Care District (HCD) of Palm Beach County is a countywide special taxing district as outlined in the 1988 Palm Beach County Health Care Act special statute, chapter 87-450, Laws of Florida. HCD's mission is to fund, plan, and coordinate health care for the medically needy and to oversee trauma services.[1] The HCD has two main objectives: (1) to fund two trauma centers in the county, and (2) to provide services for persons who do not have health insurance, which it does by administering a managed care program for uninsured persons, operating a school health program, administering a rehabilitation and nursing center, and providing local match funding for the Florida KidCare program.[2]

---

[1]See http://www.hcdpbc.org.

[2]Florida KidCare is the state's children's health insurance program.

The HCD has a seven-member, voluntary board of commissioners, three members of which are appointed by the Palm Beach Board of Commissioners, three by the governor of Florida, and one by a representative of the Florida Department of Health. Thus, the board can be held accountable to the county through the selection of the HCD board members appointed by the County Commission. HCD commission terms are four years, and commissioners are permitted to hold appointments for up to eight consecutive years.[3]

The HCD administers a managed care program, the Coordinated Care Program (CCP), for its medically needy residents who do not qualify for Medicare or Medicaid. The program funds inpatient hospital services, primary- and specialty-care services, dental services, vision care, and prescription drugs. In this program, public dollars follow the patient seeking health care services. Hospitals are reimbursed on a per diem basis, and physicians are reimbursed on a fee-for-service basis, using rates set at 80 percent of Medicare reimbursement for participating physicians and 60 percent for nonparticipating physicians.

Approximately 26,500 residents are served annually through CCP, which has an annual budget of approximately $35 million. Residents with incomes at or below 150 percent of the federal poverty level (pregnant women may have incomes of up to 200 percent of the federal poverty level) and assets of less than $10,000 for ßan individual or couple (house and car not included) qualify for the plan. CCP is affiliated with the county health department, all hospitals in the county, numerous health clinics, and 1,000 participating primary- and specialty-care physicians.[4]

St. Louis Regional Health Commission

A series of events culminating in the year 2000 motivated officials of the city of St. Louis and St. Louis County to change the way regional health care providers meet the needs of the uninsured and underinsured. The region's public health care system lacked sustainable funding, and service provision for indigent care was fragmented.[5] Moreover, since 1999, community groups had complained about the dearth of services at St. Louis's public hospital system, ConnectCare,[6]

---

[3]See http://www.hcdpbc.org.

[4]Debi Gavras, Administrator of Risk Operations, Health Care District of Palm Beach County, Florida, personal communication, February 26, 2003.

[5]Missouri Department of Social Services, "Missouri Medicaid 1115 Waiver: Health Care for the Indigent of St. Louis," submitted to The Center for Medicare and Medicaid Services, August 21, 2001, p. 3.

[6]ConnectCare is a nonprofit, public private partnership of the city of St. Louis, the state of Missouri, and four hospital systems in the region.

which faced increasing financial pressure to reduce services or close its inpatient facility. The possible closure of the inpatient facilities threatened the loss of nearly $20 million in federal DSH funds to the St. Louis area.[7] Public outcry about insufficient services and the threat of losing DSH funding prompted city, county, and state officials to convene representatives from the public health community to discuss health care access for the uninsured.[8]

In April 2000, another group concerned about the same issues, St. Louis Civic Progress (an organization of area CEOs from business sectors), established an indigent health task force. The task force included a variety of community organizations, health providers, and representatives from the governor's office, the St. Louis mayor's office, and the St. Louis County executive office. This group met to address the imminent funding crisis, to discuss how to improve care for the medically indigent, and to develop a regional plan that would reduce institutional competition among organizations caring for the underserved.

One of the task force's primary recommendations was the establishment of a St. Louis Regional Health Commission (RHC). In conjunction with the Missouri Department of Social Services (DSS), the RHC was founded in September 2001 (see Figure 4.1).[9] The mission of the RHC is to increase access to health care for the medically uninsured and underinsured, to decrease health disparities among populations in the region, and to improve health outcomes for these populations. Currently the RHC is charged with two principal tasks: (1) develop a strategic plan for provision of indigent health care services by the end of 2003, and (2) coordinate the implementation of the plan. This plan will outline "a financially sustainable system that provides quality care and access to care for all residents."[10] The RHC is expected to achieve its goals through strategic planning, communication/reporting, education, funding guidance, and community health improvement.[11]

The 19-member RHC will engage the community; distill and analyze data; research, propose, and recommend system changes; develop measures of

---

[7]The Center for Medicare and Medicaid Services allocates DSH funds based on the number of inpatient services used by the uninsured.

[8]Missouri Department of Social Services, *Missouri Medicaid 1115 Waiver*, p. 7.

[9]St. Louis Regional Health Commission, "Workplan," June 19, 2002, p. 3, available at http://www.stlrhc.org/About/Workplan.aspx (accessed January 15, 2003).

[10]Interview with Robert Fruend, CEO, Regional Health Commission, November 5, 2002.

[11]St. Louis Regional Health Commission, "Workplan," p. 4.

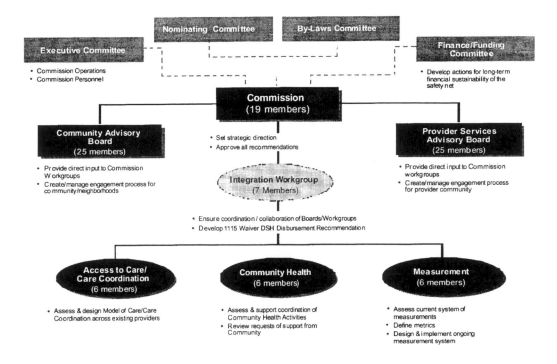

SOURCE: St. Louis Regional Health Commission, "Workplan," June 19, 2002, available at http://www.stlrhc.org/About/Workplan.aspx (accessed January 15, 2003).

Figure 4.1—Organizational Structure of the St. Louis Regional Health Commission

success; act as the chartering authority for advisory boards and work groups; and supervise work plans, budgets, and policies of the commission. The structure of the RHC is subject to change, but currently it has five committees (executive, nominating, bylaws, finance/funding, and integration workgroup), two advisory boards (community, provider services), and three work groups (access to care/care coordination, community health, and measurement). All committees, advisory boards, and work groups have between 9 and 25 members; work groups have the smallest memberships.[12] These bodies draw on a wide variety of experience and expertise, with representatives from the Department of Health, schools of public health and medicine, physicians, public insurance departments, hospital administration, community providers, community advocacy groups, and religious organizations. Formed as a result of minimal coordination among these representatives and public officials, the RHC, particularly the RHC board, has become the primary body through which these representatives work

---

[12]Ibid., pp. 8–13.

28

together.[13] Robert Fruend, the CEO of the RHC, is an *ex officio* member of every body.[14]

To support the activities of the commission, the DSS applied for and in August 2002 was granted a Medicaid 1115 waiver to direct DSH payments to the St. Louis Regional DSH Funding Authority (RDFA),[15] a nonprofit corporation consisting of the CEOs of the four major hospital systems and two major independent hospitals in the city of St. Louis and St. Louis County.[16]

The RHC receives Medicaid 1115 waiver funds only through approval and oversight of the state DSS and the local RDFA. The RHC submits recommendations to the RDFA concerning DSH funding disbursement, and the RDFA, with approval of the DSS, assures that the money is distributed according to RHC plans.[17] The RHC also supports ConnectCare, the region's public hospital system, which closed its hospital facility in November 2002 and now operates a network of clinics. The RHC receives funding for administration and staffing from the city, county, and state. The RHC staff of three has an annual administrative budget of $500,000 for five years.[18]

Looking to future sustainability, the RHC has as a goal the oversight of disbursement not only of the waiver funds but also of regionwide funds for the medically underserved. To date, the region has made little effort to coordinate funding sources. The county has its own health department, and through a dedicated tax, it operates three clinics. Additionally, in April 2001, city voters approved a 2.725-cent tax on out-of-state purchases of more than $2,000. The city dedicates $5 million of these revenues to ConnectCare.[19] Ultimately, the RHC hopes to phase out acute-care facilities and focus on ConnectCare's community clinics. Moreover, the RHC plans to distribute funding across other primary and specialty care in neighborhood clinics and to integrate the St. Louis area's health care delivery system.

Since the RHC is still in its infancy (a permanent CEO was hired in May 2002), it is too early to tell how well this new structure will address the needs of the

---

[13]Interview with Robert Fruend, CEO, Regional Health Commission, November 5, 2002.

[14]See www.stlrhc.org.

[15]This waiver was an addendum to an existing Missouri 1115 waiver. The RHC will receive funding until March 2004, when it will be required to reapply.

[16]P.J.C. Health Care; St. John's Mercy Health Care; Sisters of Mercy Health Systems–St. Louis; Tenet Health Care St. Louis; St. Anthony's Medical Center; and St. Luke's Hospital.

[17]St. Louis Regional Health Commission, "Workplan," p. 6.

[18]Interview with Robert Fruend, CEO, Regional Health Commission, November 5, 2002.

[19]*St. Louis Post-Dispatch*, July 5, 2002, available at http://Web.lexis-nexis.com/universe (accessed January 13, 2002).

uninsured and underinsured in St. Louis. Moreover, there is no guarantee that the proposed structure will endure, as the RHC is designed to be an interim step to longer-term health care system integration. Nevertheless, the RHC provides valuable lessons for policymakers seeking governance structures that reinforce accountability in the planning, coordination, and monitoring of the indigent-care system. A central coordinating body like the RHC could facilitate the bringing together of interdependent provider groups to offer indigent-care services that are more efficient and cost-effective.

Johns Hopkins Medicine

Given the growing trend of municipalities selling their public hospitals (Bovbjerg, Marsteller, and Ullman, 2000; Friedman, 1997), there are few examples of successful county-owned academic medical centers. Thus we turned to the private sector for governance models of complex medical centers. Johns Hopkins Medicine (JHM)[20] is a unique example of interorganization cooperation and coordination that is implemented through a university. JHM is an umbrella organization that encompasses the Johns Hopkins Health Care System (JHHCS), the Johns Hopkins Hospital (JHH), and two associated hospitals, Johns Hopkins Bayview Medical Center (JHBMC) and Howard County General Hospital (HCGH). Each subsidiary organization has its own board, and some officers serve on more than one board. For example, the chairman of the JHM board also serves as the chairman of the JHH and JHHCS boards. JHH and JHHCS share the same president and several corporate officers.[21] The boards of JHM, JHH, and JHHCS also share some of the same officers—one of the vice chairmen for JHM is also a vice chairman of JHH, and the president of JHM serves as an *ex officio* vice chairman of the JHHCS. The two associated hospitals have their own boards of directors, but there is some overlap of members. For example, one of the vice chairmen of JHM is a vice chairman of the JHBMC. Similarly, the chairman of the board of HCGH serves as an *ex officio* member of the JHM board.

The interlocking boards show consistency with the principles of governance discussed in Chapter 3 of this report. The three principal Johns Hopkins facilities (JHM, JHHCS, and JHH) have the same board chairman, which allows consistency of communication across organizations at the board level. The president of JHM is an *ex officio* member of the boards of JHHCS and JHH, again

---

[20]Institutional information is available at http://www.hopkinsmedicine.org.

[21]Specifically, the two organizations share vice presidents for corporate services, planning and marketing, facilities, human resources, general counsel, operations integration, and management information systems.

supporting communication among the organizations. However, importantly, the boards of the physical entities (JHHCS, JHH, JHBMC, and HCGH) all have 15 or fewer members, which enables them to work efficiently.

While this example presents the interrelationships among organizations associated principally through a university connection, there are some general observations to be made. First, the boards of directors of the various physical organizations are fairly small, having 15 or fewer members. Second, functionally related organizations have one or two overlapping members. Third, while the board of the umbrella organization is too large,[22] according to the recommendations of Carver or Pointer and Orlikoff, the executive committee has 17 members and in all likelihood functions as the primary connection between the board and the president/CEO.

Summary

The Health Care District of Palm Beach County operates a managed care program for indigent county residents in which the dollars follow the patient and which allows for good accountability of services and public expenditures. The St. Louis RHC exemplifies an innovative governance structure for coordinating care for the uninsured and for dispersing DSH funds that provides opportunities for input from owners, stakeholders, and the community in general. Finally, Johns Hopkins Medicine features well-structured governance boards for a complex academic medical center and affiliated institutions.

None of these governance structures is necessarily replicable in Miami-Dade County. However, policymakers and public officials in Miami-Dade can draw on the examples during their deliberations about the design and operation of an integrated model for health care services for the uninsured. In the following chapter, we turn to indigent health care in Miami-Dade and the related governance challenges.

---

[22]The JHM Board of Directors has 52 members.

5. Miami-Dade County Public Health Trust

The Miami-Dade County Public Health Trust (PHT) currently has a $1.3 billion annual operating budget with which it operates a complex of health care services institutions ranging from primary-care clinics to secondary- and tertiary-care facilities;[1] long-term-care nursing and correctional health facilities; and managed care programs through the Jackson Health Plan. As the county government-owned health system in Miami-Dade, the PHT provides the majority of hospital care to the county's nearly half-million uninsured residents. The principal hospital in the system, Jackson Memorial Hospital (JMH), in partnership with the University of Miami, is one of the largest academic medical centers in the nation. For some specialties, the hospital ranks among the nation's top 25 institutions.[2]

Before looking at the current governance structure of the PHT and assessing it in terms of the governance principles outlined in Chapter 3, we present a brief history of the organization since its inception in 1973. Much of this discussion draws on our earlier report, *Hospital Care for the Uninsured in Miami-Dade County: Hospital Finance and Patient Travel Patterns* (Jackson et al., 2002).

History of the PHT

Before the Half-Penny Surtax

The PHT was created in 1973 by the Miami-Dade Board of County Commissioners (BCC) to govern JMH, the county's government-owned hospital. The PHT's authority was described in County Ordinance 73-69:[3]

---

[1]Primary care is oriented toward the daily, routine needs of patients (such as initial diagnosis and continuing treatment of common illnesses) and is provided in outpatient facilities. Secondary care includes "routine" hospitalization and specialized outpatient care. Tertiary care includes the most complex services (such as open heart surgery, burn treatment, and transplantation) and is provided in inpatient hospital facilities.

[2]For example, JMH is one of the top 25 hospitals in the nation in treating eye disorders; one of the top 25 in pediatrics; and one of the second 25 in gynecology and treatment of kidney disease, ear-nose-throat disorders, and digestive disorders (2000 *U.S. News and World Report* hospital rankings, February 9, 2001, update, available at http://www.usnews.com/usnews/nycu/health).

[3]Section 9 of Ordinance 73-69 was adopted July 30, 1973, and codified as Chapter 25A, Public Health Trust, of the Miami-Dade County Code.

32

> The board of trustees shall have the powers, duties and responsibilities customarily vested in trustees and, to the extent consistent therewith, shall also have the powers, duties and responsibilities customarily vested in the board of directors of a private corporation.

From its inception, the PHT was given the governance role for JMH akin to that of any corporate board of directors.

The PHT was (and still is) accountable to the BCC and, by extension, to the county populace. Initially, the BCC was involved in the selection of PHT trustees, with trustee nominations made by the Health Systems Agency (HSA). Three nominees for each vacancy were forwarded to the BCC, permitting choice in their selection. This process has changed, as discussed below.

The hospital was also accountable for the amount of charity care provided. Hospital management submitted to the county management detailed billing statements for all indigent-care patients treated at the facility. While the county often did not reimburse the hospital fully for the care provided, there was a clear link between the care provided an indigent patient and the public dollars used to pay for that care.

The Half-Penny Surtax

The late 1980s and early 1990s were particularly difficult years for the hospital industry. The growth of health maintenance organizations, competition among hospitals, and the increasing number of uninsured caused many hospitals to run into financial difficulty. To alleviate some of the financial stresses associated with uncompensated care, the state of Florida in 1991 passed legislation permitting local taxing districts to hold referenda for approval of tax levies to finance health care for the indigent.[4] The 1991 Florida Surtax Statute required counties to continue to fund county hospitals to the extent of at least 80 percent of the prior county funding, in addition to any surtax levied. This support was labeled the maintenance-of-effort (MOE) requirement.

In September 1991, Dade County voters approved a sales surtax of 0.5 percent, the proceeds of which were earmarked "for the operation, maintenance and administration of Jackson Memorial Hospital to improve health care services."[5]

---

[4]Title XIV, Taxation and Finance, Chapter 212, Tax on Sales, Use and Other Transactions. For Miami-Dade, the law assigned surtax revenues to the sole public hospital, without restricting the revenues to the provision of care to the indigent. The surtaxes applying to other large counties and to small counties were designated for indigent care, not for the local county hospital.

[5]Language from the referendum ballot.

At the time the tax was initiated, JMH was operating at a loss. The infusion of funds helped stabilize the hospital's finances and expand the role of the PHT.

With the infusion of funds from the surtax, the relationship between the PHT and the BCC changed. First, the PHT no longer reported detailed claims for indigent patients to the BCC. We do not have a transcript of the discussion, but we assume that the BCC funding that provided MOE support and surtax revenues acted as a block grant to the hospital to cover these costs. Second, rather than having some health care facilities directly under the BCC, the BCC moved correctional health and two long-term-care nursing facilities into the PHT budget. Third, in the expansion of the PHT's role, the BCC expected that the PHT would be responsible for oversight of the planning for health care services for the entire county. This new role is articulated in Article III, amended purposes (a) and (c). Specifically,

> The purpose(s) of the Trust shall also include:
>
> (a) Participation in activities designed to promote the general health of the community;
>
> (b) Fulfillment of the objectives set forth by the Commission in the Trust Ordinance and compliance with County-wide health care delivery policies which have been or may be established by the Commission.

While the majority of PHT facilities were located in the urban areas of Miami, the PHT was expected to provide care to any county resident who did not, for whatever reason, have access to health care services. The BCC's mandate to the PHT required it to consider expansion of publicly supported services into heretofore less-served areas. The BCC also expanded the PHT's board from 15 to 21 voting members. To provide diversity and inclusiveness, the BCC required that the 21 members reflect various professions or segments of the Miami-Dade community.[6]

While the surtax accomplished the goal of providing additional funds to JMH, thereby enabling continuation of its role as the county's public hospital, JMH was not the only health care provider serving the uninsured. By 1993–1994, other hospitals in the Miami-Dade County area that cared for the indigent began to

---

[6]No more than two members from law, banking and finance, public accounting, corporate management, education and business; one each with public health and professional nursing expertise; one from the University of Miami Board of Trustees; one officer of the Miami-Dade Medical Association; one governing board member from a local nonprofit hospital; one governing board member of a local, private nonprofit primary-care center; three members among the indigent users or organizations serving the indigent population; and one member from the disabled community. These requirements have since been eliminated.

voice concerns that they deserved a share of the surtax revenue.[7] These other facilities argued that they were more cost-effective than JMH and, because of their geographic location, would allow patients to receive care closer to their homes (Guber, 1993).

There has been considerable controversy surrounding the original intent of the surtax and, in particular, the governance of the funds provided by it. Two main assertions are that (1) the administration, planning, and evaluation of the surtax funds' use should be accomplished by an independent board, i.e., one that is not connected to a provider of services, as is the case with the PHT and JMH; and (2) many uninsured persons live substantial distances from JMH but must travel to JMH for their hospital care, bypassing numerous other hospitals. We address each of these assertions below.

An Independent Body for Planning and Evaluation. At the same time the surtax was passed, an indigent health care task force was convened to consider the health care needs of the uninsured. This task force recommended in 1992 that, among other things, the county "establish an independent board that would plan, control financing and monitor the indigent health care system."[8] However, when the Miami-Dade County Health Policy Authority (HPA) was created in 1995 (Miami-Dade County Ordinance 95-71), it was required to advise the BCC through the PHT (Hoo-you, 2000)—i.e., all HPA recommendations and reports to guide BCC policy had to go through the PHT for review before being submitted to the BCC for approval. This even included any plans the HPA might recommend for incentive programs "to encourage private providers to provide uncompensated health care services to the indigent residents of Miami-Dade County" (Miami-Dade County Ordinance 95-71, Article LXVI, Section 2-436).

In addition to this reporting structure, one-third of the HPA's board members are also PHT board members. This lack of independence created "a perception that the Trust was filtering reports and not moving forward on reports submitted by the Authority."[9] The PHT later moved to rectify this by passing a resolution requesting that the HPA simultaneously submit all reports to the PHT and to the BCC. However, the PHT retained the authority to request that the reports become items on the BCC agenda where they are acted upon.

Several attempts have been made over the past few years to revise the ordinance of the HPA, to make it a fully independent entity, accountable to the BCC, that

---

[7]Nancy Ancrum, member of the editing board of the *Miami Herald*, personal communication, 2001.

[8]Report of the Dade County Indigent Health Care Task Force, 1992.

[9]PHT Board of Trustees meeting minutes, December 14, 2000.

could plan and evaluate indigent health care across the county. One recommendation for change was made by Commissioner Barreiro, who proposed an HPA ordinance revision that would make the HPA report directly to the BCC and would reconfigure its board to make it more independent of the PHT (Hoo-you, 2000). In addition to changing the reporting mechanism for the HPA, Barreiro's proposal would have formally created dialogue between the HPA and the PHT regarding health care planning in the county. However, to date, the HPA remains inextricably linked to the PHT and therefore cannot independently develop health care policy for the county.

Geographic Access to Care. The surtax funds are allocated to the PHT, which has its major hospital facility in the northeastern, more-urban area of Miami-Dade County. Most of the other hospitals in the county are also located in the densely populated northeastern area, leaving the western and southern areas with fewer facilities providing care for the uninsured and, until very recently, no other hospital funded with surtax dollars.[10] The centralization of publicly funded hospital facilities has led to disparities in geographic access to hospital care between the uninsured and the insured (Jackson et al., 2002) and is a continuing cause for concern among some activists and policymakers.

Partly in response to these concerns, the Florida Legislature, on May 5, 2000, amended the Florida Surtax Statute to make it possible for providers other than the county hospital, JMH, to receive county funding for indigent health care (the Florida Surtax Amendment). Known as the Lacasa Bill (HB71, 2000), this amendment proposed to divert up to 25 percent of the county's MOE funding to a special fund, to be administered by a board independent from that which runs the county public hospital, so that all eligible hospitals within the county could make claims against this fund for reimbursement in proportion to the uncompensated care they provided. This amendment would have transformed the Miami-Dade County system into one in which some of the dollars followed the patient. However, on September 19, 2000, the Miami-Dade BCC declared through Ordinance 00-111 that this amendment violated Miami-Dade County's Home Rule Charter and refused to comply with it. As a result, several hospitals filed a lawsuit on February 8, 2001, to require the county to implement the Surtax Amendment (and thereby remit the required funds to an independent authority to fund a plan for indigent health care services). The lawsuit was dismissed without prejudice on July 24, 2001. The private hospitals filed an amended complaint on September 26, 2001, which has also since been dismissed.

---

[10]The Public Health Trust purchase of Deering Hospital, subsequently renamed Jackson South Community Hospital, added a facility in South Dade. We discuss this in more detail later.

Concern about access to hospital care by the indigent in South Dade arguably moved the PHT to action.[11] As early as 1998,[12] the PHT entered into negotiations with HCA–Columbia for the purchase of Deering Hospital, a community hospital in South Dade. In 2000, negotiations with Deering were stalled, and Homestead Hospital, a major provider of charity care in South Dade, approached the PHT and asked it to take over Homestead's operation, allowing the infusion of surtax funds to offset losses from the increasing indigent population in the area. Negotiations went on for several months but eventually ended when the PHT and Baptist Health South Florida, Homestead's parent corporation, could not find a mutually satisfactory solution. Baptist was willing to have the PHT operate Homestead Hospital, but it wanted to retain ownership.

When negotiations with Baptist/Homestead fell through, the PHT looked again to Deering Hospital, which it purchased in June 2001, renaming it Jackson South Community Hospital (JSCH) (McNair, 2001).[13] Under the PHT's umbrella, JSCH could benefit from its association with JMH and also have access to surtax dollars. Coincidentally, negotiations with Deering's parent company, HCA, were undoubtedly eased, as HCA agreed to sell the hospital as part of a settlement of federal fraud charges.

In sum, through the 1990s, the Miami-Dade County PHT grew, and its board of trustees assumed responsibility not only for governing the operation of an increasing number of facilities, but also for developing policies and means to provide health care to the county's indigent residents. This dual mission made certain activities difficult. Reflecting on the Homestead and Deering negotiations, some people questioned whether the PHT could work with other health care providers to provide care to all county residents, particularly the uninsured (Dorschner, 2002; Garwood, 2002).

The Current Situation

The Mayor's Health Care Access Task Force

Seeking direction and solutions to the problem of the uninsured, Miami-Dade County Mayor Alex Penelas created a health care access task force in February

---

[11]Our earlier report showed that South Dade has a large uninsured population, many of whom travel from South Dade to JMH for their care, often bypassing closer hospitals.

[12]As indicated in the PHT Board of Trustees meeting minutes, June 11, 1998.

[13]JSCH is 20 miles south of JMH, providing geographically close access to care for uninsured persons living in the rural area of South Dade. The Jackson Health System Strategic Plan (Lewin, 2001) estimates that JSCH will free up 24 beds at JMH, as patients from South Dade will travel to JSCH rather than to JMH.

2002 to examine the county's health care system. The task force was directed specifically to look at options for expanding health insurance coverage to the working uninsured, to identify ways to improve the existing delivery system and resources, to explore coverage alternatives, and to examine issues of governance, planning, and organization. The task force created subcommittees to address these four issues and was scheduled to make final recommendations in March 2003.

Current PHT Reporting Structure

The PHT is accountable to the Miami-Dade BCC and, by extension, to the residents of the county. The PHT reporting structure is shown in Figure 5.1.

The BCC created the Health Policy Authority to conduct health policy planning. The HPA, in turn, contracts with other nonprofit agencies such as the Health Council of South Florida to produce analyses and reports. Some would argue, however, that the true role of the HPA is unclear (and "compromised" (Hoo-you, 2000)), as its recommendations are considered by the PHT before they are passed on to the BCC. To further complicate the process, both the HPA and the PHT are required by ordinance to confer with each other in the development of a single, countywide five-year strategic plan.

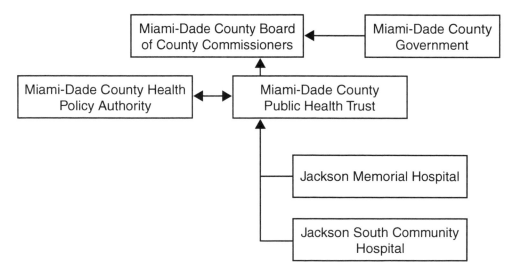

Figure 5.1—Current Reporting Structure of the Public Health Trust and Health Policy Authority

Current PHT Governance Structure

Candidates for the PHT board are nominated by a council appointed by the mayor, and the nominations are ratified by the BCC. Trustees serve three-year terms that can be renewed three times, for a total of nine years. Terms of individual trustees are staggered to allow for continuity. Trustees may be removed by a majority vote of the BCC. The current PHT board consists of 21 voting members and eight *ex officio* nonvoting members (three county commissioners, the county manager or his or her designee, the president of the PHT, the senior vice president for medical affairs at the University of Miami, the president of the JMH medical staff, and the dean of the University of Miami School of Medicine). Thus, the PHT board has a total of 29 members.[14]

The PHT conducts business under bylaws that specify responsibilities and structure. These bylaws follow a traditional structure and adhere, for the most part, to the principles outlined in Chapter 3.[15] They can be modified by the board itself, with approval by the BCC following. They have been modified 25 times since 1973. The BCC can also modify the PHT's role through its ordinance-writing authority.

Over time, the bylaws have been made more specific as issues have arisen. For example, in 1999, the bylaw committee added a limitation on the number of consecutive years an external auditor may be used.[16] Missing, however, is the clear articulation of board policy and active monitoring. This long-standing lack of action has, unfortunately, created problems.

A Critical Look at PHT Governance

Thus far, we have identified two important problems in the current governance structure of the PHT that have contributed to a decline in the public's trust of the system: (1) the dual role of the PHT creates an inherent potential for conflict of interest, and (2) the transparency and accountability in the actions of the PHT and the way the surtax funds are used have deteriorated.

In addition to these two broad issues, our analysis of the governance of the PHT identified some specific areas where changes should be considered. Some examples of missed opportunities for board action and ambiguity in the bylaws

---

[14]This composition of the board differs from the previous structure, in which the 21 voting trustee positions were designated by specific demographic characteristics. The BCC recently eliminated the population-segment-specific rules for board membership.

[15]Most recent revision of the bylaws, dated February 2, 1999.

[16]Article VIII, Section (2)(b)(11).

are discussed below. These examples do not constitute a complete catalog of issues; rather, they are meant to be illustrative.

Missed Opportunities for Board Action

CEO. The board has the authority to appoint, evaluate the performance of, set compensation and benefits for, and, if necessary, remove the president of the PHT. Unfortunately, the board has not been performing these important functions. Information revealed during the events surrounding the resignation of PHT President Ira Clark in November 2002 indicated that the board had not conducted a performance review of the CEO for several years, nor had it reviewed his salary for the previous five years. Without such an evaluation, it is unclear how the PHT was able to effectively monitor the organization for which it is responsible.

As stated in the bylaws, the compensation committee, which is responsible for making recommendations to the board concerning CEO compensation, is effectively a subcommittee of the executive committee.[17] The bylaws provide no provision for an explicit connection between CEO performance and compensation. Moreover, the compensation committee structure makes it vulnerable to political considerations. The seven voting members of the committee include the mayor or his or her commissioner-designate and a commissioner appointed by the mayor. Unlike the bylaws specifying other committee membership, those concerning the compensation committee do not specify that the commissioners who are members need to be board members as well.

Board Member Tenure. The bylaws are clear with respect to the length and number of terms an individual member can serve. However, there appears to be no rigorous monitoring of or appreciation for the benefit of board turnover. Recently, the member who held the seat designated for the University of Miami resigned after having served 12 years on the board. While it is important to have continuity in board membership, excessively long tenure can breed familiarity that ultimately diminishes objective oversight.

Board Member Attendance. The bylaws state that members must not have more than three unexcused absences from regular board meetings or three unexcused absences from committee meetings. A two-thirds vote of the board is required for a member who misses five board or committee meetings to remain on the

---

[17]Article VIII, Section (5).

board. A review of the minutes for the past several years revealed that in both 1998 and 1999, two board members had five absences, yet one of them was reappointed the following year. There is no evidence in the board minutes that the members with absences exceeding stated thresholds were acknowledged, nor is there evidence of board action to retain members with excessive absences, although such action is required by the bylaws.

Currently, the minutes include individual meeting attendance, but there is no distinction between excused and unexcused absences, as required by the bylaws,[18] nor is there any cumulative reporting of absences to alert the board to potential problems.

Committee minutes presented in PHT board meeting agenda packets also show that there were numerous times when quorums were not reached. The PHT attendance problem was discussed by the BCC's Health, Public Safety, and Human Services Committee on May 15, 2002. It was proposed that disinterested members be replaced with competent, qualified individuals, but action was deferred when one commissioner questioned the ethnic and gender composition of the board and requested that a report be provided to the BCC.[19]

Follow-Through on Board Requests. The minutes reveal that there is no consistent reporting of follow-through on board requests to management. Without such follow-through, it is difficult for the board to hold management accountable. A retrospective study of minutes showed that board members have frequently posed the question, "Whatever happened to [a particular issue]?"— suggesting that there was no follow-through or closure.

Another example of apparent lack of board follow-through with management is the perennial request by the county's Office of the Inspector General (OIG) to have an office at the PHT from which to conduct business. The minutes document the general lack of space at the medical complex, but they also document that retail space has become available from time to time. The minutes do not reflect any discussion of the costs and benefits of using such available space for auditors, nor do they directly address the board's policy or management's actions concerning the OIG's concern about internal control procedures at the PHT. Indeed, there has been resistance on the part of the board to address this issue.

---

[18]A board discussion on September 10, 1998, resulted in requiring members to provide a written request for an excused absence 10 days in advance of a meeting. However, since that date, no unexcused absences have been noted in the minutes.

[19]Miami-Dade Legislative Item File Number 021067.

To facilitate tracking board member requests, the board could adopt a comprehensive calendar of board meetings and committee and subcommittee meetings with such requests appropriately annotated. Moreover, such a calendar would provide board members and the public the opportunity to become further informed. A review of the committee minutes as distributed in the agenda packet indicates that there are numerous opportunities for board member education when staff present overviews of programs to committee members. Notification of scheduled meetings would provide the opportunity for others to become familiar with the organization.

Ambiguity in the Bylaws

Board Orientation and Self-Evaluation. The PHT is responsible for orienting, educating, and periodically evaluating the board and its members. Particular attention has been paid to the issues of quality of care and quality assurance, but there appear to be few opportunities for additional board member training on governance issues. Moreover, the bylaws do not include specific requirements for board retreats, nor do they give the board chairman the authority to influence the content of the educational material provided to board members. The bylaws should be revised to give the board more control over its work, orientation, education, and training.

Composition of the Board of Trustees and Potential Conflicts of Interest. The PHT is a public entity, yet a significant number of board members are from the University of Miami, a private institution that provides the medical staff to the PHT's hospitals and is thus a customer of the PHT. Specifically, one voting member seat on the board is reserved for a University of Miami trustee, and the dean of the University of Miami School of Medicine is a nonvoting, *ex officio* member. Nonvoting, *ex officio* positions are also reserved for the senior vice president of medical affairs and the president of the PHT medical staff. If either of these individuals has University of Miami connections, the potential for influence is considerable. The business relationship between the PHT and the university should be specified through the annual agreement that serves as a contract between the two entities, rather than through any possible influence on the PHT board.

As discussed in Chapter 3, board members have the clear responsibility to consider the needs and wishes of owners and stakeholders and to make decisions that are best for the organization. When stakeholders are also customers, there is the potential for conflict of interest in making those decisions. Moreover, it has recently been revealed that the agreement between the PHT and the University of

Miami has never been audited. Even in the absence of true conflict of interest, the lack of transparency in the relationship erodes public trust.

Committees and Subcommittees of the PHT. A number of standing committees of the PHT are specified by the bylaws. These include the executive committee, the fiscal affairs committee, the joint conference committee, the program planning and primary-care committee, the facilities development committee, and the personnel and labor relations committee. In addition, the committee structure includes an officers nominating committee, a quality improvement committee, a compensation committee, and a strategic planning committee. In contrast to the recommendations of Carver (2002) and Pointer and Orlikoff (1999, 2002a,b), the bylaw descriptions of some standing committees are ambiguous as to the distinction between board policymaking and oversight authority and management activity. This ambiguity can potentially cause problems if management staff feel compelled to report to board committees rather than to the CEO.

Because the committee structure is set explicitly in the bylaws, there is little incentive for the board to review its committee structure to determine what committees should be convened to address the issues that must be considered in the upcoming time period. As previously suggested, it is important that a board thoughtfully consider the work that needs to be done and the best way to do it. While the bylaws give the chairman the authority to create special committees[20] and have them ratified by the board,[21] there appears to be no way for the board to disband a committee specified in the bylaws when it is no longer necessary.

PHT Progress Toward Better Governance

Many of the observations that we have made regarding shortcomings in the governance of the PHT have been noted before. Numerous efforts to effect change from outside the PHT have failed, and recommendations have met with resistance or have fallen on deaf ears. Recently resigned PHT Chairman Michael Kosnitzky made a concerted effort in his short tenure to move the PHT to better governance. Perhaps he made his push for reform too quickly, and not all board members were committed to his suggested changes. Therefore, his tenure as chairman was cut short by a vote of the board. The new chair will have to work to achieve consensus and resolve to continue moving the PHT to active governing rather than passive monitoring.

---

[20]Article VIII, Section (1)(e)(f).
[21]Article VIII, Section (1)(i).

Summary

At its inception, the PHT was responsible for governing only one institution, JMH. Today, some 30 years later, it is responsible for a countywide system of facilities for the indigent, as well as for planning, delivering care, and evaluating access countywide. However, its governance structure has remained largely the same: The same board has oversight over the county-owned health care facilities and over the development and monitoring of countywide health care policy. As additional responsibilities have been given to the PHT by the BCC, its bylaws have been modified. However, the modifications have introduced ambiguity, potential conflicts of interest, and the potential for political influence. Moreover, recent history has shown numerous instances where the board has not acted in accordance with its bylaws. This lack of action undermines accountability and transparency, eroding public trust.

Community-led efforts to separate the planning, financing, and evaluating of indigent care from the delivery of services have had mixed results. The ordinance creating the HPA and its resulting governance structure have prevented it from acting as a fully independent planning body, and efforts to revise the ordinance to make the HPA fully independent have been unsuccessful. State legislation to create an independent board to administer a portion of the PHT's MOE funds for countywide indigent care was blocked by local county commissioners and was ultimately found by the court to be in violation of Florida's Home Rule Charter. The fact that the mayor's health care task force, convened in 2002, identified governance, planning, and organization as a priority demonstrates that the issue remains of considerable concern to local providers, activists, and policymakers.

6. Discussion and Conclusions

The PHT clearly sees its role as that of a public provider of health care services. It is responsible for oversight of the medical complex comprising Jackson Memorial Hospital (JMH), Jackson South Community Hospital (JSCH), associated clinics, and other care facilities, and it has an operating budget of more than $1 billion. In addition, it has the responsibility for planning for the health care needs of the entire county's indigent population. Thus, if we ask, What is the PHT governing?, the answer is the dual mission of service provision and countywide planning—a situation that inherently introduces a conflict of interest: Is the best governance structure for the PHT the best governance structure for an organization responsible for health care policy planning for the entire county?

The answer to the question, For whom is the PHT governing?, is equally problematic. Under its current governance structure, the PHT reports to the BCC. But reviews of BCC and PHT minutes suggest long-standing communication and reporting problems between the two bodies. Indeed, members of the BCC have commented that they did not feel the PHT was sufficiently accountable to them.[1] If the PHT is not held accountable to the BCC, can the public find the PHT accountable?

These issues, while problematic, do not diminish the significant contributions the PHT has made to the residents of Miami-Dade County. JMH is world-renowned and well respected. It holds a very important position in Miami-Dade County, as a health care provider and also as a major employer. However, because the health services delivery component of the PHT has grown considerably in the past decade, this function should now have its own discrete governance structure.

Under the current ordinance structure, two public entities are involved in publicly funded health care issues, the PHT and the HPA. The PHT's inherent conflict of interest is a compelling reason to move all policy development and analysis from the PHT to the HPA. In making this change, the respective missions of the PHT and the HPA would become clearer and there would be no

---

[1]The BCC met in a workshop on May 5, 2001, to discuss Commissioner Moss's recommended amendments to the PHT ordinance for improved governance, to include "the preparation of any report requested by the Commission to be delivered within 30 days of such request; and presentation of quarterly financial reports to the Commission" (Miami-Dade Legislative Item File Number 010129).

conflict of interest. Indeed, such a change would allow the PHT to connect more directly with its owners and stakeholders. Similarly, the HPA could connect with the county's populace to ascertain the broader perspective needed for countywide policy and planning.

In the remainder of this chapter, we present our recommendations for separating service provision and countywide policy and planning. Our recommendations are informed by what we learned about governance structures elsewhere. The system adopted by Palm Beach County, where the dollar follows the patient, facilitates accountability by enabling the HCD to report the numbers of persons served, the types of services they received, etc. The governance structure for planning and policy in St. Louis provides opportunity for community input. And we learned from examining Johns Hopkins Medicine that complex organizations may find it useful to consider decentralizing governance. We incorporate each of these lessons in our recommendations.

Admittedly, implementing some of the recommendations would require fundamental change, but legislative language is already in place that would allow for implementation of most of them. Some recommendations relate to administrative matters that would improve the transparency and accountability of both the PHT and the HPA. The ultimate decision about whether or not to accept and implement the recommendations rests with the mayor, the BCC, and Miami-Dade County residents. Collectively, they must decide how they want their local government to plan for the county's health care needs, how the public funds dedicated to health care should be spent, and how to make the health care system more accountable and transparent in discharging its responsibilities to the public.

Recommendations Requiring Fundamental Change

Our primary recommendation is that the county policymaking role be separated from the service provision role; both are currently under the governance of the Miami-Dade County PHT. We recommend that the countywide health care policy component be realigned and renamed the Health Policy Trust (HPT) to reflect its new countywide mission and responsibility. Because the PHT has become synonymous with the Jackson Health System, we recommend that the governing body for the Jackson Health System and JMH be named the Board of Trustees, Jackson Health System (BTJHS). We offer these names as mere suggestions, but we do recommend the change of names to clarify purpose and to signify that a change has occurred. Our proposed structure is illustrated in Figure 6.1.

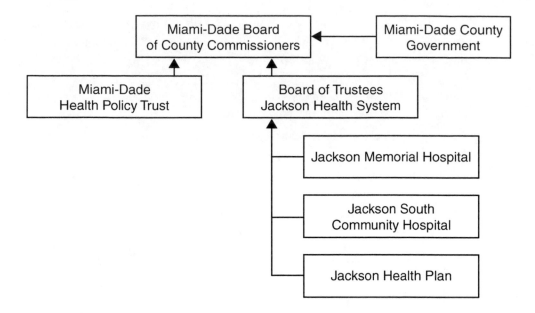

Figure 6.1—Recommended Governance Structure for Miami-Dade County Health Care Policy and Provision

This is a propitious time to make these changes. The president of the PHT, Ira Clark, was asked to resign in November 2002 (after this report was requested and Mayor Penelas convened the health care task force). Then, in December 2002, PHT Chairman Michael Kosnitzky announced his resignation effective April 2003. He was subsequently voted out in February 2003. Both resignations put the PHT clearly in a transition that presents opportunity for change. This opportunity was succinctly summarized by the mayor when he wrote to the PHT:

> Moreover, it is critical that the responsibilities of the new President be clearly defined. Whether the new President will be in charge of the County's *entire* health care system or of operating Jackson Memorial Hospital, or both, is a basic policy issue. These are among the prevailing health care issues currently being discussed by the members of Mayor's Health Care Access Task Force. The timing for this community debate could not be more appropriate but it must occur before the search process comes to a conclusion [emphasis added]. (Penelas, 2002)

Effecting this change requires changes in structures as well as processes. In the following, we discuss recommendations for change in the various governing bodies.

The Miami-Dade County Board of Commissioners

The BCC has legal oversight of the PHT and the HPA, but it is clear that this oversight has not been executed effectively. We recommend that the BCC consider carefully whether or not it needs to have oversight of the new HPT and the BTJHS.

If the BCC is to continue exercising oversight, then it is incumbent upon it to require that the governing bodies it oversees make regular, formal presentations and/or reports. These reports should provide accountability and transparency, documenting statistics that relate to services and processes consistent with the respective missions of the institutions. Working with the governing boards, the BCC can design effective reporting mechanisms that are not duplicative and that provide the necessary information to permit effective oversight.

The mayor and the BCC should carefully consider ways to keep the HPT and BTJHS apolitical and focused on their respective missions. Any undercurrent of political influence contributes to the detriment of transparency and hence reduces public trust in these important public institutions.

However, it can be argued that the BCC need not continue to oversee these activities directly; rather, the HPT and the BTJHS could be independent bodies. Each could report to the BCC in an advisory manner, providing the opportunity for the public to be informed. The BCC could continue its role in selecting board members, but we suggest that selection follow explicit guidelines to maintain boards with diverse experiences and skills sets. This would support transparency, accountability, and local input—all features of good governance.

The Board of Trustees, Jackson Health System

The BTJHS would govern all of the various health services facilities that are part of the county-owned integrated system. Because the system is very large, the BTJHS should consider creating a decentralized governance structure for its subsidiary organizations, i.e., JMH, JSCH, and the Jackson Heath Plan. The various boards could have interconnected membership as required, although, adhering to the principles of the policy governance model, the number of members in common should be limited to two or fewer.

Regardless of whether a centralized or decentralized governance structure is established, we recommend that the size of the board be reduced to permit more effective governance. Ideally, the board should have nine to 19 members, and its composition should be carefully determined to avoid potential conflicts of interest. The number of inside board members should be limited, consistent with the principle that no more than 25 percent of the board should be insider or *ex officio* members. Organizations that have both common and vested interests, such as the University of Miami, should not have voting representatives on the board. The university could communicate with the new governing board through the annual negotiation of their shared services agreement. This relationship would more clearly define the roles of the board, management, stakeholders, and customers. As such, the shared services agreement could be structured to provide more transparency and accountability, and it should be audited periodically.

As the Jackson Health System moves forward, its new board will also have to consider once again the question of governance for whom. As discussed in its strategic plan, JMH requires, for its financial viability, that it provide care to both the indigent and the insured, both publicly and privately. The board will need to clearly specify performance goals to ensure that there is no competition for resources that diminishes appropriate treatment and service for either customer group.

The Health Policy Trust

We recommend that the HPT be Miami-Dade County's principal health policymaking body, communicating directly with the Miami-Dade County BCC in making policy and implementing recommendations. This new reporting relationship would require modification of the ordinance. However, our reading of the record suggests that these changes are consistent with the original intent.

As part of its mission, the HPT should elicit input from the community. One effective way to generate public visibility is to hold regularly scheduled town hall meetings where different groups in the county can present their health care needs and priorities. The HPT should develop mechanisms for input that are culturally appropriate, that are convenient for community members, and that encourage participation. This input should be considered integral to policy development.

In sum, with this proposed structure, the relationship between planning for and delivery of services becomes more transparent. In developing its five-year plan for the county's health care needs, the HPT should consider the facilities of the Jackson Health System among the rest of the county's health care resources. This would enable it to consider opportunities to work with other health care providers to improve access to care for residents and to consider cost and quality in its policy calculus. As additional funding for services is made available, the

HPT would be able to consider cost-effectiveness and quality in its negotiations with providers in a way that is impossible under the current sole-source arrangement. If appropriate, the HPT should contract with providers outside the Jackson Health System to improve access for the uninsured in various parts of the county.

With this new organizational structure, the board of the HPT should be reconstituted and expanded. Currently, three HPA board members are also PHT board members. We suggest that the new board of the HPT have independent members. As a policymaking body, the board should comprise individuals who can understand the issues and think broadly and fairly. Moreover, the HPT should consider the myriad of potential trustees among business leaders, school administrators, and welfare advocates.

Funding Concerns

Throughout our examination of indigent health care in Miami-Dade County, an overriding concern has been the future fiscal viability of the PHT and the Jackson Health System. This concern was articulated by the past PHT president numerous times, especially when anyone raised the issue of collaborating and sharing the surtax with other hospitals serving the uninsured. Clearly, the Jackson Health System will remain a major player in the health care system of the county and will continue to provide tertiary and trauma care, two activities that benefit the entire populace, are expensive, and are often regionalized.

Before the HPT can make changes, it will have to take an inventory of the county's health care resources and needs, a task that will undoubtedly require more staff to provide analysis and interpretation. To work effectively, the HPT will have to carefully consider various models to engage staff with the essential skills for its new mission. Furthermore, the HPT will want to work collaboratively with state-funded and other-funded agencies that are already performing some of this inventorying of resources and needs.

Numerous organizations in Miami-Dade County are involved in health care policy and planning, and many are funded to some degree with county dollars. For example, in addition to the HPA and the PHT, the Health Council of South Florida and the Alliance for Human Services have also received funding from the county to do health planning and related activities. The BCC should consider consolidating the health planning activities and associated funding streams of these and other publicly funded organizations and redirecting the funding and activities to the HPT.[2] These funds would provide a start-up allocation for the HPT in its new role as the primary health planning agency for the county. Of course, the new HPT may want to contract out for services during a phase-in period as they develop the knowledge and capacity to perform these activities and deliver the services outlined. Moreover, in consolidating funding, the county will have to consider various matching and leveraging opportunities so that no funding is lost.

Such start-up funds, however, will not be sufficient to carry out the planning and evaluation of countywide health care, nor will they enable the HPT to design mechanisms to directly fund care for the uninsured. It has been estimated that more than $1.3 billion would be needed to provide insurance for the 450,000 uninsured county residents.[3] However, these calculations do not take into account the amount that is currently being used to provide care to this population by JHS and other providers. It is thus unclear what additional funding would actually be required to set up a countywide system that could serve the indigent with a broader, more geographically dispersed set of reimbursed providers. Moreover, actually implementing a health plan for the uninsured goes well beyond a planning role and requires the capacity to allocate funding, monitor, and evaluate program processes and outcomes.

The HPT would need the commitment of additional funds to effect change in how and where the uninsured get health care. There are several funding strategies the county might consider. First, it could reallocate existing tax-based funds to the HPT. This may seem difficult, given the hold that the current PHT has on revenue from the half-penny sales tax and property taxes. However, there is a precedent for considering the diversion of some of these resources. When the PHT was considering the implications of the Lacasa Bill (HB71, 2000), it approved a resolution that would have diverted some of its MOE funds to a new, independent health authority. Specifically, the resolution proposed that the PHT divert to the new authority $10 million in year 1, $15 million in year 2, and $21.9 million in years 3 through 5.[4] Miami-Dade County was to provide matching funds, meaning that in the first five years, the new independent health authority

---

[2]By consolidating, we do not mean that these other organizations should cease to exist. We are recommending, however, that public funds for health care planning activities should be directed to the county body responsible for this (HPT). Cutting the pie into so many pieces means that no one agency can do much of anything, and establishing aggregate accountability ifor the totality of funds and objectives can be challenging..

[3]This estimate is based on the calculation of 450,000 uninsured × $3,000 for a prepaid managed care plan such as the Jackson Health Plan or Trust Care.

[4]Resolution PHT 04/00-051, described in the PHT minutes for April 26, 2000.

would receive more than $180 million. This proposed funding could be directed to the new HPT to provide funding for an indigent-health-care plan (or plans).

In addition to reallocating existing tax funding, the HPT and county might consider additional tax-based strategies. For example, they could propose election measures to assess additional property taxes or an additional half-penny sales tax to fund the HPT, which could then develop mechanisms to reimburse more providers of health care services to the uninsured. Specifically, the HPT could consider creating a system similar to that of Palm Beach County, in which the dollars follow the patient.

Raising taxes during the current economic and political climate may seem difficult. Yet in Los Angeles County, an area facing significant fiscal challenges, voters in November 2002 approved a ballot proposition that raised property taxes three cents per square foot (about $42 for a 1,400-square-foot house) to provide additional funding for emergency rooms and trauma centers. The proposal passed with well over the two-thirds majority required and earned more support than any other measure or candidate in the county (Richardson and Ornstein, 2002).

Finally, to further its policy development and implementation role, we recommend that the HPT be given the authority to secure grant and contract funding (such authority is not explicitly included in the ordinance language). Much innovation in the health care arena is funded by foundations such as the Robert Wood Johnson Foundation and the W. K. Kellogg Foundation and by federal agencies such as the Health Resources and Services Administration. Being able to access these funding sources would provide additional opportunities for the HPT. Moreover, the HPT should become a leader in innovation regarding expansions of Medicaid and other federal-state programs. Such expansions often provide the opportunity to leverage funds through matching. Building a diverse funding base for health care for the uninsured and underinsured would provide needed stability for patients as well as providers.

Administrative Change Recommendations

We offer several administrative recommendations that should improve the transparency and accountability of both the HPT and the BTJHS under any governance structure that is ultimately put in place in Miami-Dade County.

Improve Accessibility of Meetings

Under Florida's sunshine rules, meetings of public entities are open to the public. While the PHT board can meet in the commission chambers, per county ordinance, and can have the meetings televised, this has not happened. Instead, meetings are held in the boardroom at JMH, which does not have video or audio equipment installed. The PHT announced in January 2003 that it would use microphones in board meetings so that the audience of staff and visitors could better listen to the discussion (Ricker, 2003a). It is important to monitor follow-through on this commitment. The public's access to the meetings has been discussed for over two years, with no result.[5] Indeed, as of February 2003, the PHT members were surprised to learn that the original Miami-Dade County Ordinance, Chapter 25A, required them to have televised meetings (Ricker, 2003b). We recommend that similar video and audio requirements apply to HPT meetings as well.

Improve Accessibility of Information

Both the HPA and the BTJHS should maintain websites where they can post institutional information such as their mission statements and board composition. Board members should be listed with their professional affiliations to provide transparency. The HPT and the BTJHS should regularly post meeting minutes, annual reports, special reports, etc. In particular, once the boards establish their annual plans and objectives, they should post performance indicators so that the public can also assess how well its public institutions are working. Access to this information would provide more transparency and accountability to the organizations' activities.

Accountability and transparency would also be increased if the HPT and the BTJHS reported "milestone" checklists on their websites. Both have clearly defined deliverables—meetings and reports—specified in their enabling legislation. The checklist would provide a mechanism for listing all these deliverables and recording when they have been completed.

Document and Report Board Member Attendance

Board and committee members could be held accountable by annotating individual member attendance with the number of meetings attended and

---

[5]The ordinance proposed by Barreiro recommended that the meetings be televised.

missed and the number of excused absences. This would allow the public and various constituencies to follow the involvement of board members. Such information would also help the boards in their self-assessments.

Report Policy-Meaningful Statistics

The boards should consider developing meaningful performance statistics and requesting that they be reported. Whether the BTJHS has one, two, or three boards, information relevant to the organization's mission should be reported clearly.

The current PHT duly receives and reviews information on hospital finance and performance statistics in the form of traditional balance sheets and operating statistics such as patient admissions, outpatient visits, etc. However, there are no statistics that relate to the hospital's provision of care to the indigent. Currently, it is impossible to discern the extent to which specialized tertiary services are used by the indigent or by insured patients. It would be helpful and would enable the board to actually monitor the institution with respect to compliance with its mission if management had to report statistics on activities of *policy* interest such as the number of uninsured persons treated in the clinics, in the ER, and in the hospital, the number that were undocumented, etc. These data are available and are reported occasionally, as revealed in a newspaper article:

> Jackson Memorial Hospital spent $51 million caring for 6,600
> undocumented and 3,300 legal foreign nationals living in Miami-Dade
> County in fiscal year 2001, part of the $300 million the hospital spent caring
> for people who could not reimburse the institution. (Chardy, 2002)

Having such information reported to the boards and the public would facilitate transparency and accountability. We recommend a similarly meaningful reporting process for the HPT. Ideally, it would compile and publish such information for all Miami-Dade hospitals.

Depoliticize the Appointment and Removal of Trustees

Currently, only one nominee per vacancy is submitted to the BCC for approval.[6] This is insufficient to assure an apolitical appointment, and it reduces the ability

---

[6]Ordinance 25A.3.d.

of the BCC to assure a diverse board.[7] The original proposal whereby three names per vacancy were submitted should be considered.

Summary

We recommend that the PHT and the HPA be realigned and renamed to reflect their respective missions. To assure that the HPT has authority within the county, we recommend that funding come from its current MOE allocation according to the compromise language agreed upon by the PHT when it was deliberating the implications of the Lacasa Bill (HB71, 2000). In making this funding recommendation, we are mindful of the current fiscal constraints at JMH. However, what is important is that the HPT be providing sufficient funding to implement change. Moreover, we recommend consolidation of the funding streams for the various health policy and planning activities currently conducted in the county. This realignment is consistent with the enabling legislation and could easily be adopted. With funding from the county as well as through contracts and grants secured from other sources, the HPT should be able to develop an integrated system of care using JHS and other providers to assure access to care for all Miami-Dade County residents. Depending on the success of its efforts, the county should consider proposing an additional tax to be used for contracted services provision. Finally, both the BTJHS and the new HPT should consider implementing some of our recommendations concerning administrative matters. This would improve the transparency and accountability of the activities of both governing bodies and their respective organizations.

---

[7]Diversity here includes, per the ordinance, reflection of the community's racial, gender, ethnic, and disabled make-up, but also the array of skills and experience needed by the board in the conduct of its work.

Appendix
The Sixty-Four Principles[1]

1. The board realizes that it alone bears ultimate responsibility, authority, and accountability for the organization. It understands the importance of governance and undertakes its work with a sense of seriousness and purpose.

2. The board understands those factors that affect governance quality and employs a coherent set of principles to govern.

3. The overarching obligation of a board is ensuring an organization's resources and capacities are deployed in ways that benefit its stakeholders. The board serves as their agent, representing, protecting, and advancing their interests and acting on their behalf.

4. The board identifies the organization's key stakeholders.

5. The board understands stakeholder interests and expectations.

6. The board decides and acts on behalf of stakeholders; it discharges its legal fiduciary duty of loyalty.

7. The board discharges its legal fiduciary duty of care.

8. The board understands the functions it must perform in order to meet its obligations.

9. The board understands and accepts its ultimate responsibility for determining the organization's ends and ensuring it has a plan for achieving them.

10. The board formulates the organization's vision.

11. The board specifies key organizational goals.

12. The board does not become directly involved in developing organizational strategies; it delegates this task to management.

13. The board understands it is ultimately responsible for ensuring high levels of executive performance.

14. The CEO is the board's only direct report.

15. When a vacancy occurs, the board selects the CEO.

---

[1]Reproduced from Dennis D. Pointer and James E. Orlikoff, *The High-Performance Board: Principles of Nonprofit Organization Governance,* Copyright © 2002, John Wiley & Sons, Inc. This material is used by permission of John Wiley & Sons, Inc.

16. The board has a CEO succession plan.

17. The board specifies its key expectations of the CEO.

18. Annually, employing explicit criteria, the board assesses the CEO's performance and contributions.

19. Annually, the board adjusts the CEO's compensation.

20. Should the need arise, the board is willing to terminate the CEO's employment.

21. The board understands that it is ultimately responsible for ensuring the quality of the organization's services or products.

22. The board has an explicit and precise working definition of quality.

23. The board develops a panel of quality indicators.

24. The board ensures the organization has a plan for improving quality.

25. The board understands it is ultimately responsible for the organization's financial health.

26. The board specifies key financial objectives for the organization.

27. The board ensures that management-devised budgets are aligned with financial objectives, key goals, and the vision.

28. The board develops a panel of financial indicators.

29. The board ensures that necessary financial controls are in place.

30. The board is ultimately responsible for itself—for its own performance and contributions.

31. The board understands that to govern effectively it must execute three core roles: policy formulation, decision-making, and oversight.

32. The board formulates policies regarding its ultimate responsibilities.

33. The board makes decisions regarding matters requiring its attention and input.

34. The board oversees (monitors and assesses) key organizational processes and outcomes.

35. When it meets, the board spends the majority of its time performing its policy formulation, decision-making, and oversight roles.

36. The board acts only collectively; and once it does so, members support its policies and decisions.

37. The board has an explicit, precise, coherent, and empowering notion of the type of work it must do—its responsibilities and roles.

57

38. The board recognizes the importance of governance structure that is consciously designed based on explicit principles, criteria, and choices.

39. Governance structure is streamlined.

40. Unless there are extraordinarily compelling reasons to do otherwise, board size ranges from nine to nineteen members.

41. If governance structure is decentralized, the authority, responsibilities, and roles of parent and subsidiary boards are explicitly and precisely specified.

42. If advisory bodies are employed, their functions are clearly specified and differentiated from those of governing boards.

43. The board specifies the roles of committees and its relationship to them.

44. The number and type of committees are designed to reflect the board's responsibilities and facilitate and support its work.

45. The functions and tasks of committees are specified by the board and codified in a charter and work plan.

46. Governance structure is thoroughly assessed at regular intervals and modified if necessary.

47. The board proactively designs and manages its composition.

48. Members are recruited and selected on the basis of explicit criteria, employing a profiling [sic, of skills] process.

49. New board members participate in a carefully crafted and executed orientation process.

50. The board specifies member expectations.

51. The board has fixed term lengths and limits the number of terms members can serve.

52. The board periodically assesses the performance and contributions of every member; the results are employed to coach and develop members and make composition redesign decisions.

53. Board composition is nonrepresentational.

54. The CEO is a voting *ex officio* member of the boards.

55. Insiders and those servicing *ex officio* comprise less than 25 percent of the board's membership.

56. The board has its own budget.

57. The board has adequate staff support.

58. The board formulates annual objectives.

59. Meeting agendas are carefully devised plans for deploying the board's attention and time.

60. Board meetings are managed and conducted to promote high levels of effectiveness, efficiency, and creativity.

61. The chair is carefully selected, understands the role, and is able to perform it effectively.

62. The board is serious about continuous member development and has a plan for accomplishing it.

63. The board should hold periodic retreats.

64. The board engages in a periodic self-assessment and formulates action plans to improve its performance and contributions.

References

Agency for Healthcare Research and Quality. *Health Insurance Coverage in the U.S. Civilian Non-Institutionalized Population, First Half of 2001*, Rockville, MD: Agency for Healthcare Research and Quality, July 2002, available at http://www.meps.ahrq.gov/CompendiumTables/01Ch1/TC01Ch1_TOC.htm.

Annison, M. H., and D. S. Wilford. *Trust Matters: New Directions in Health Care Leadership*, San Francisco, CA: Jossey-Bass, 1998.

Bovbjerg, R. R., J. A. Marsteller, and F. C. Ullman. *Health Care for the Poor and Uninsured After a Public Hospital's Closure or Conversion: Assessing the New Federalism*, Washington, DC: Urban Institute, Occasional Paper Number 39, 2000.

Carver, John. *On Board Leadership: Selected Writings from the Creator of the World's Most Provocative and Systematic Governance Model*, San Francisco, CA: Jossey-Bass, 2002.

Carver, John, and M. Carver. "Carver's Policy Governance Model in Nonprofit Organizations," available at http://www.carvergovernance.com/model.htm (originally published in French in the Canadian journal *Gouvernance: Revue Internationale*, Vol. 2, No. 1, Hiver 2001).

Chardy, Alfonso. "Foreign Visitors Burden Hospitals," *Miami Herald*, January 8, 2002.

Dorschner, John. "Better Cooperation Envisioned for Jackson," *Miami Herald*, November 22, 2002.

Friedman, Emily. "California Public Hospitals. The Buck Has Stopped," *JAMA*, Vol. 277, No. 7, February 19, 1997, pp. 577–581.

Garwood, John. "New Leadership Needed for Miami-Dade Public Health Trust," Editorial, November 25, 2002, available at http://www.click10.com/.

Greenleaf, Robert K. *Servant-Leadership: A Journey into the Nature of Legitimate Power and Greatness*, New York: Paulist Press, 1977.

Guber, Susan. "For Better Health Care, Make Better Use of What Dade Has," *Miami Herald*, November 24, 1993, p. 13A.

Hebert, Robert. "For Struggling States, All Solutions Point to Washington," *The New York Times*, December 2, 2002.

Hoo-you, Hilary J. *A Historical Compendium of Miami-Dade Health Care Planning Initiatives: A Decade Report*, Miami, FL: Miami-Dade County Health Policy Authority, March 30, 2000.

Jackson, Catherine A., Kathryn Pitkin Derose, James R. Chiesa, and Jose J. Escarce. *Hospital Care for the Uninsured in Miami-Dade County: Hospital Finance and Patient Travel Patterns*, Santa Monica, CA: RAND, MR-1522-CH, 2002.

Kearns, Kevin P. *Managing for Accountability*, San Francisco, CA: Jossey-Bass, 1996.

The Lewin Group, *Jackson Health System Strategic Plan: Building a Health Care System for Miami-Dade County's Future*, final report pending Public Health Trust Board of Trustees approval, 2001.

Los Angeles Times. "Unhealthy Push for Profit," Editorial, November 22, 2002, p. B18.

McAdam, Terry W., and David L. Gies. "Managing Expectations: What Effective Board Members Ought to Expect from Nonprofit Organizations," in David L. Gies, J. Steven Ott, and Jay M. Shafritz (eds.), *The Nonprofit Organization: Essential Readings*, Pacific Grove, CA: Brooks/Cole Publishing Co., 1990, pp. 189–197.

McDonough, William J. "Issues in Corporate Governance," *Current Issues in Economics and Finance*, Vol. 8, No. 8, September/October 2002.

McNair, James. *Miami Herald*, June 22, 2001, p. 1-C.

Miami-Dade County Code of Ordinances. Ordinance 73-69, Chapter 25A, Public Health Trust, available at http://www.municode.com.

Miami-Dade County Code of Ordinances. Ordinance 95-71, Article XLVI, Miami-Dade County Health Policy Authority, available at http://www.municode.com.

Moore, Stephen. *Proposition 13 Then, Now and Forever*, Washington, DC: Cato Institute, July 30, 1998, available at http://www.cato.org/cgi-bin/scripts/printechn.cgi/dailys/7-30-98.html.

Penelas, Alex. Letter to the Public Health Trust, December 11, 2002.

Pointer, Dennis D., and James E. Orlikoff. *Board Work: Governing Health Care Organizations*. San Francisco, CA: Jossey-Bass, 1999.

Pointer, Dennis D., and James E. Orlikoff. *The High-Performance Board: Principles of Nonprofit Organization Governance*, San Francisco, CA: Jossey-Bass, 2002a.

Pointer, Dennis D., and James E. Orlikoff. *Getting to Great: Principles of Health Care Organization Governance*, San Francisco, CA: Jossey-Bass, 2002b.

Public Health Trust By-Laws. Public Health Trust of Miami-Dade County, Florida, Jackson Memorial Hospital, Miami, FL.

Richardson, Lisa, and Charles Ornstein. "Hospital Funding Plan Passes. Partial Returns Show Ballot Measure for L.A. County Medical Facility Has Two-Thirds Majority. Museum Upgrade Plan Falls Short," *Los Angeles Times*, November 6, 2002.

Ricker, Daniel A. *The Watchdog* , Vol. 3, No. 33, January 13, 2003a.

Ricker, Daniel A. *The Watchdog*, Vol. 3, No. 38, February 17, 2003b.

Roper Center at the University of Connecticut. *Public Opinion Online*, poll taken early September 2002, available at http://web.lexis-nexis.com.

Salamon, Lester M. "The New Governance and the Tools of Public Action: An Introduction," 28 *Fordham Urb. L.J.* 1611, 2001.

Schooner, S. L. "Fear of Oversight: The Fundamental Failure of Businesslike Government," 50 *AM. U.L. Rev.* 627, February 2001.

Strom, Stephanie. "Questions Arise on Accounting at United Way," *The New York Times*, November 19, 2002.

Webster's Encyclopedic Unabridged Dictionary of the English Language. New York: Portland House, 1997.

Winter, Greg. "School Learns Cost of a Gift-Giver's Anger: Case Western University and Peter B. Lewis," *The New York Times*, November 14, 2002.